"If they awarded Purple Hearts to people with Crohn's disease, Audrey Kron would have one by now. A veteran of more than 30 hospital stays and many operations, Kron is a psychotherapist who uses her experience to help people cope with Crohn's disease and ulcerative colitis. 'Good reading can be a gateway to good health,' notes Kron. Ask Audrey is a case in point."

Barbara Rosenstein
CCFA Foundation Focus

"Audrey's positive, open approach to all aspects of IBD is inspiring, and her wisdom and insight, born of her own struggles with the illness, shine through on every page. The result is that her readers are encouraged to be challenged by the disease rather than defeated by it. Ask Audrey is recommended reading for all who live with IBD and those who work therapeutically with them."

Judy Sobczak
Michigan Women Psychologist Network

"Information and assuring describes Ask Audrey. Audrey Kron's book answers the questions everyone who lives with IBD wants to know. Sharing how others cope with day-to-day problems and anxieties is the strength of this book."

Oley Foundation

"She takes the confusion out of dealing with hospitals, doctors, tests and treatment; as well as more common issues like controlling pain or just getting out of bed in the morning. In fact, the problem doesn't have to be IBD and the reader doesn't have to be ill. The book is good for everyone—it was a joy to read and easy to understand. And the opportunity to make your own notes along the way gives a sense of participation. Bottom line: you no longer feel alone."

Esther Liwazer
Michigan CCFA Newsletter

"If readers struggling with IBD share concerns or questions tackled here by Kron—diarrhea, sexuality or Total Parenteral Nutrition (TPN), for example—they will find a wealth of common sense and inspiration in her answers, drawn from Audrey's own experience and research. I would venture to suggest that there is probably a gem of wisdom or enthusiasm for every reader to draw inspiration from, especially those readers living with IBD."

Peter McGinn
Ostomy Quarterly

"This well-written book is the result of a lifetime of living and learning with IBD by Audrey Kron, a woman who has gone through the best and worst of Crohn's disease. I recommend this book for patients and people interested in IBD because it does cover a number of questions generally not answered in textbooks or brochures."

Dr. Micheline Ste-Marie
Education Chair
Medical Advisory Board
Crohn's & Colitis Foundation of Canda

"Although the book deals with Inflammatory Bowel Disease, the information is useful for many illnesses."

Carla Jean Schwartz
Detroit Jewish News

"The depth of feeling and poignancy in Kron's responses set this book apart from others of its type. The wisdom in this work is exemplified by such gems as, 'Start now to make IBD just a passenger, not the driver in your life.'"

Fred Zeller
Better Together Now Bulletin

Also by Audrey Kron, M.A.

Meeting the Challenge:
Living with Chronic Illness

Ask Audrey

The Author's Personal and Professional Experience in the Day-to-Day Living with Inflammatory Bowel Disease

Audrey Kron M.A.

Hints on taking control of illness rather than letting it control you

ASK AUDREY, Sixth Printing
Copyright © 1992, 1994, 1998 by Audrey Kron

ISBN: 0-9633877-0-7
Printed in the United States of America

Cover design by Doug Braunschweig
Layout by Rick Broida, Elizabeth Pernick

 This book was printed using recycled paper.

ACKNOWLEDGEMENTS

This book is the result of a lifetime of living and learning. However, it could not have been accomplished without the help of some very special people. Thank you hardly seems adequate, but I do want to acknowledge:

- My supportive family and wonderful friends for being there.

- Edith Broida for her editing, encouragement and empathy.

- Sylvia Bartlett, Debbie Lundy and the staff and volunteers at the office of the Michigan Chapter CCFA who made this book a reality.

- Jason Bodzin, MD, for reading the manuscript for medical accuracy.

- Lois Hutchinson, RN, Caroline Trapp, RN, Marion Cashero, Judie Rosen, Silvana DeSanto, Esther Liwazer, Donna Ryan, Sharon LaCasse, Ilene Karson and Rick Broida for their assistance.

- I would especially like to thank my readers, my clients and the many individuals with IBD whom I have known. From them I have learned what courage and determination can accomplish.

PREFACE

Dear Readers,

   I would like to share with you some of my thoughts about the composition of this book. In the beginning I struggled with delving into my own personal story, especially since I am in a profession that usually requires some anonymity. I ultimately decided that it would be valuable for you to know that the comments in this book aren't just from text books. They also represent years of the trial and error of living with IBD as well as working professionally with individuals and family members dealing with chronic illness.

   This book is not a medical book. The ideas expressed aren't necessarily CCFA's responses or those of any particular physician or institution. However, I have consulted with many professionals to convey as accurate a picture as I can. The IBD experience is different for every individual. Do not take what I say as the final word. Instead, use my ideas to stimulate your thinking. If you have questions, consult with your doctor. What was helpful for me, in some cases, may not work for you.

   Most of the questions and answers originally appeared in my "Ask Audrey" column in the Michigan Chapter CCFA Newsletter. They have been edited for this book.

   The format of the book allows each section to stand on its own, therefore there is some repetition. I left it that way so that you may return to an individual column when the situation applies and you won't have to refer back and forth to other columns as frequently to obtain the information you want.

   When the book was blocked out, there were empty spaces between the columns. At first, I thought of eliminating the blank areas. Then I decided to retain them to enable you to have the space to add your own responses or personally relevant ideas. I find that during difficult times, even I go back to my own columns for help. If you personalize each article, you, too, will have something to turn to when necessary.

So, I'm asking you not only to read this book, but, in some way, to start writing your own. Clarifying my thoughts on living with IBD has made an important difference in my life. I hope that it will be as beneficial to you!

CONTENTS

PART I:
MY STORY

I have few memories of being sick as a child. I do remember chicken pox. I sat on the front porch blowing bubbles out of a bubble pipe...and shared my toys. Soon the whole neighborhood had chicken pox.

Next I remember having what the doctors thought was whooping cough. We had been at our summer cottage and had to pack everything to take home so I could be near the doctor. Nothing about the whooping cough comes to mind; however, I do remember the trip from the cottage. I had insisted that we take my pet turtles home with us, much to my mothers's chagrin. During the journey the tomatoes and the bed linens fell into their tub of water. My mother would have gladly dispensed with the turtles, but I was insistent that they stay.

Later, when we returned to the cottage, I left their tub outside, and it rained. The water rose, and two of the three turtles crawled off to the lake. I felt the third turtle would be lonely, so I freed him as well. That is all I can remember about illness until I was 16.

At 16 I had my first experience in the hospital, an emergency appendectomy. I had no idea what to expect. On the way home I told my father that now at least I knew what to take with me if I ever returned. He just said, "Shhh," as if that would keep me from ever passing through the hospital doors again.

"Shhh" wasn't enough. That episode was just the beginning of well over 30 hospital stays. The hardest part of my appendix operation was trying not to laugh. Laughing hurt - and the frequent paging for what sounded like, "Dr. Baked Beans" didn't help.

At 17 my health hadn't improved. Later we were to realize that the appendix operation had just been the result of a misdiagnosis. My high school drama teacher, Mr. White, was the first person to actually recognize how sick I was. He had cast me as Elizabeth Barrett in "The Barretts of Wimpole Street." Saying "Doctor, doctor," as I lay on the couch didn't require acting. Soon

I was in the hospital again for more testing. I never did get to play the role. Thirty years later I was able to make up for that disappointment and take part in a production of "Fiddler on the Roof."

My medical tests in Detroit proved futile. The doctors still had no idea as to why I was in so much pain and growing weaker all the time. They considered mononucleosis, but seemed tentative in their diagnosis. My family decided to make a pilgrimage to the Mayo Clinic.

In 1954 the Mayo Clinic was the mecca for any type of illness. People came from all over to find some hope. For many, it was the last resort. Most patients stayed in hotels and scheduled various tests and treatments as out-patients. The restaurants in the area had become accustomed to seeing patrons with all kinds of medical problems. For example, one day I passed out at the table, and without even blinking the waitress brought a cold compress and continued to serve our table.

Before long I was admitted to the hospital at Mayo because I was running a fever. That was an experience. Only the sickest were confined to the hospital. Because our insurance did not cover an out-of-state hospital, I decided against a semi-private room and entered a 12-bed ward. In the end bed lay Charlotte, who prayed aloud all day. Her body was encased in a neck-to-body cast, and she roller-skated in place to exercise her legs. Despite her own difficulties, she was quite supportive. Across the way was a country woman who kept a black satchel filled with food hidden under the bed. Periodically she would sneak under the bed for some forbidden nourishment. There was also Molly who wandered around with a bag of fluid hanging down, which was totally unfamiliar to me at that time. There were constant moans and screams. All in all, it wasn't the kind of place a 17-year old would like to spend her summer vacation.

Each day the doctors would find some new diagnostic tool. One day I had to have the bone marrow test. I already knew that this had to do with leukemia. It was extremely painful. I had particular difficulty with this procedure because of a previous experience in Detroit, in which an intern had asked, "Is this the right instrument to use?" My confidence had been shattered. Later I watched mothers in the waiting room preparing young children for what lay ahead. I still have a vivid picture of one mother talking to her son. He had looked so worried, but when the nurse called, he lifted his head and just bravely marched in.

That night at Mayo, after the bone marrow test, the intern stopped by my bed. I asked for the results. It had been routine to tell me that each test had been negative. This time the intern said in a solemn voice that they wanted to talk to my mother in the morning. I was sure that I had a terminal illness: leukemia.

Soon my mother arrived, but I didn't share my concern and told her to go to the movies. I felt there was no sense in both of us worrying. That night I was sure I was going to die. I thought of how I wanted to spend my last days. The next morning the doctors came, and said that they had figured out that I had ulcerative colitis. It was another misdiagnosis (later, they were to find out I had Crohn's disease) but, at that time, I was so excited that I would live, I didn't care what it was I had.

We returned home shortly after. The long drive was difficult. I was so weak that I could hardly walk, let alone climb stairs. I also had terrible diarrhea so we had to find restaurants with lavatories on the first floor. Because I was so sick, I would often just abandon my food so that we could leave. Another complication was that the inactivity in the hospital had led to phlebitis. The pain was so intense that when we stopped at my aunt and uncles's house on the way home, I couldn't be moved any further. The following week just getting to the bathroom was an ordeal.

I graduated high school with difficulty. It wasn't that I had trouble with my studies, but I did have trouble with my energy. Just climbing stairs was overwhelming. In particular, I remember Miss Harnack. Everyone thought that she was mean, but often she would let me rest instead of going to class, and she allowed me to stay upstairs when they had practice fire drills.

When graduation day rolled around, everyone was worried about whether I would be able to walk across the stage to accept a scholarship award. I believe I had been given a Chrysler scholarship because I had a deeper awareness of the meaning of life than did most 17 year-olds. I made it across the stage, but when the students marched out, I didn't have enough energy to go back with them.

Despite the illness, I had become very involved in the B'nai B'rith Youth Organization. I served as chapter president and then as Michigan Regional president. When the elections for regional officers took place, I had just had my appendix out and wasn't able to climb stairs. My best friend Jeanie found a young man to carry me up the stairs. Later, both he and I were installed respectively as regional presidents for AZA and BBG (part of the B'nai B'rith Youth Organization). That's how I met the man that was later to become my husband.

Larry and I worked together in BBYO, and dated. Then he went off to the University of Michigan. During that time, and for years to come, there were frequent hospitalizations. During one such hospital stay, Larry came in for the weekend and visited me at the hospital. I suggested that he date other girls because I wasn't available for the normal dating activities. He just said that as far as he was concerned we were going steady. That was just the beginning of the many times we would spend together in the hospital. More important though, it was the beginning of a marriage that is still going strong.

But I'm getting a little ahead of my story. I had been advised by my high school counselor not to go to college because it would be too difficult physically. Nonetheless, with scholarship in hand, I registered at Wayne University (now Wayne State University). Again just getting to and from class was harder than the classes themselves.

One day I fell down in the snow and couldn't walk any farther. Some workmen picked me up and asked where I wanted to go. I pointed to my classroom, and they brought me there. The teacher, who was becoming accustomed to my passing out, just said calmly, "Who wants to take Audrey home today?"

I became adept at planning around my illness. I knew that if I got sick in the middle of the term, I could convince the teacher to let me make up the work. However, I knew that if I became sick in the beginning, it was hopeless. I also became quite expert at negotiating with the expediting committee. I had to schedule my classes based on their location. If they weren't close together, I knew I couldn't make it.

Just getting to school was an ordeal. I didn't have a car so I either took the 45-minute bus ride or arranged transportation. I remember feeling so weak standing in the cold to catch a bus. But I just kept plugging away. During this period I had had my first intestinal surgery. At that time medical practice dictated the early removal of inflamed sections of the intestine. Then, I believed that the surgery would eliminate the Crohn's disease.

Despite everything, Larry and I were able to get married in 1956, and shortly after we moved up to Ann Arbor. Larry was already in law school but I was still working on my undergraduate degree. I was proficient in finding classes according to location, but the Crohn's disease wasn't as easy to plan. The frequent hospitalizations slowed me down. I even tried taking correspondence courses one semester when I couldn't manage getting to classes. As hard as I tried, I still wasn't done with my undergraduate work when Larry finished law school. I encountered endless red tape but finally managed to finish my work at Wayne University and still earn my degree from the University of Michigan.

Larry landed a job in a law firm in Detroit. At that time beginning lawyers were asked if they had an additional income since the wages were so low. We were happy to be receiving any income. As students we had been budgeting every last nickel. A Saturday night pizza was a big treat.

My degree was in education. I had wanted to be a psychiatrist but most girls at that time became teachers. It had been such a long struggle; I expected the bands to play and the earth to stop for just a minute. However, since it had taken so long, there was no one I knew in my graduating class. So the news of my graduation came very unceremoniously in a letter from the University. Inwardly the bands did play and I felt I had achieved a real victory. I was also five months pregnant.

Our son Michael made his debut at Sinai Hospital in Detroit. My obstetrician, Dr. David Feld, had been extremely cautious during my entire pregnancy. At one point I had wanted to go out on a boat, and he remarked dryly that I could only if it were anchored. I couldn't really blame him. There was some question as to whether I should even get pregnant, and additional concerns about whether I could deliver a healthy baby. It had been decided that I would have a Caesarian section. I was actually looking forward to it. I wanted once in my life to walk into the hospital with my makeup on, my hair done, and in street clothes. I was accustomed to being rushed into emergency, when how I looked was my least concern.

As it turned out, Michael came earlier than the expected date. I didn't even realize I was in labor that night. I had been used to a lot of pain with the IBD (Inflammatory Bowel Disease). I had heard women talking about labor pains and thought this new pain would be much worse. Just in case, I did get out of bed and started folding laundry. When the pains were a few minutes apart, I woke Larry and we called the doctor. He wanted me at the hospital immediately, so I still didn't get my dream of going to the hospital "like a lady."

During Michael's early years, I was a wife and mother. I did volunteer work and took classes, but I felt I couldn't do anything that required a regular schedule. I was in the hospital so often that Michael built hospitals instead of houses when he played with his blocks. At that time I kept a suitcase packed since I had become a regular at Sinai Hospital. Larry once sent me a card addressed to "Audrey, Sinai Hospital, Detroit" with nothing more on the envelope, and it was delivered to me.

At this time I developed a fistula, and nothing seemed to heal it. Dr. Fredrick Coller, an Ann Arbor surgeon, suggested three surgeries to alleviate the problem. I had already been through several resections and was not looking forward to more surgery. I discussed the surgery with Dr. Myer Teitelbaum, my internist.

Dr. Teitelbaum was a wonderful man. He has since died, but he was the epitome of what a doctor should be. He made me feel good the minute he entered my room. I also called him my booking agent. He was always willing to admit that someone else might have more information. Consequently, I came in contact with many wonderful doctors. Dr. Coller, who has also since died, was among them. I had confidence in both of them and went ahead with the triple surgery plan.

The first surgery was an ileostomy (the diversion of fecal waste through a surgically created opening of the ileum to the body wall. Waste collects in an appliance attached to the skin by special adhesive). At that time there wasn't the information available that there is now. The ostomy group in Detroit was run by Tillie Bieman, a long-time ostomate who operated the only ostomy organization in Michigan from her home.

I'd like to be able to say that having the ostomy was a breeze. Years later, when I had my second ostomy, the situation was much different. But in those early years it was a real struggle. Tillie was helpful in teaching me the mechanics. At that time there weren't stoma therapists.

As soon as I was able, I became involved in the local ostomy group and served as president for several years. In that capacity, I was instrumental in arranging a scholarship that enabled the first stoma therapist to be trained in Michigan. I dreamed of having a stoma therapist in every hospital, and today that dream is almost a reality.

I had the ostomy for about a year; and the next stage was to correct the fistula. The second operation accomplished this. Then the doctors wanted to eliminate the ostomy. By this time I had become used to it and questioned the decision, but I yielded to the medical opinions and the ostomy was reversed.

This turned out to make my life much worse. I had no control, and accidents became a way of life. In addition to the accidents, I had to deal with the prednisone that had become the new favored treatment for Crohn's disease. My condition did improve, but the puffiness and the hair growth were difficult to accept. There was also the uncertainty of additional side effects.

During these years I had been in the hospital over 30 times. After 30 I stopped counting. There were times that I spent whole seasons in the hospital. I knew how they celebrated every holiday and what special treats I could expect on my dinner tray. Many times we would rush to emergency. One time Larry asked the doctor when I would be able to come home and he said, "Don't ask 'when': ask, 'if'."

Another time I was suffering from an electrolyte imbalance and passed out. When I came to, I saw my family standing around the bed. I became alarmed when I saw my Uncle Harry. I knew he hated to come to the hospital. The first words out of my mouth were, "Uncle Harry's here. They think I'm dying." (After that I could never convince him that I understood his reluctance coming to the hospital. He became a frequent visitor).

Even the hospital staff were becoming accustomed to my frequent visits. I tried to keep my life as normal as possible despite the interruptions. One resident physician, Bill Sills, came to my hospital room because he wanted to meet "the person who conducted bridge tournaments from her hospital bed." We didn't know it then, but later Bill and his lovely wife Michele would become our very good friends.

I made a real effort to make my hospitalizations as pleasant as possible, a definite challenge. I would decorate my room with pictures and cards. I would establish a support system with other patients and hospital staff. Finally I would try to carry on my social life by inviting friends to visit and arrange for refreshments. It was different, but possible. Granted there were days that just turning over was a major endeavor. I just did the best I could.

During this time my sister was also diagnosed with Crohn's disease. Today we immediately consider IBD if a sibling presents gastrointestinal symptoms. But at that time, however, she had to endure numerous tests to determine a diagnosis. I had been out of town when she was finally hospitalized. As soon as I returned, I rushed right to the hospital. The first words out of her mouth were, "Audrey, you're a saint." I had no idea what she was talking about. She continued, "I used to visit you in the hospital and you made it look like it was so much fun. It's not fun at all!" Subsequently Judie, too, learned how to make the most out of her bouts in the hospital.

Despite the constant difficulties with my illness, I still managed to be a wife and mother, do volunteer work, travel, work on a research team, play tournament bridge, and start a women's literature group. This group still continues as an important support system for me.

In the mid-1960's I had a miscarriage. During that period, many children still needed homes. My husband and I decided to adopt, and Bob, at age three months, became our second son. It was right after the assassinations of Robert Kennedy and Martin Luther King. Robert Martin Kron was named for both men, with the hope that his future would hold less violence.

Bob was an active child, and there were days that I wondered if I would have enough energy to last until Larry returned home from work. The love for each other and for our sons was so strong, though, that we decided that we would adopt another child in a few years.

I was the traditional wife and mother of our generation. But the world was starting to change. I had just read Betty Friedan's *Feminine Mystique* and was reading Germaine Greer when Larry had to go out of town for a seminar. I decided that would be a good time to ask a single friend over for dinner. Carol said that she was now seeing someone and asked if Jim, a fellow social worker, could come as well. In my traditional view, I would have waited until Larry returned, and then arrange to get together. However, with this new "liberation" I thought, "Why not?" This may not seem like much now, but in those days we were *very* traditional.

At dinner adoption became a topic of conversation. A short time later, Jim heard of a mother that was looking for a good home for her baby, and again we became parents. This time it was a daughter whom we named Karen Elizabeth.

We had previously signed up for an additional child with Oakland County Children's Aid Society, where we had adopted Bob. But we had been so busy that we hadn't been aware of the changes taking place in our society. Abortion had become legal, birth control was more accepted, and single mothers were keeping their babies. After we decided to take Karen, we started receiving calls from couples wanting to know how we found our baby. I'm known as the kind of person that would gladly give up something of mine to help someone less fortunate. However, there was a bonding that took place with Karen the moment we decided to adopt her. We could no more give her away than we could Michael or Bob.

With three children and the many activities in which I was involved, the years flew by. We continued to try to keep everything as normal as possible, and I searched for ways to cope with my limited energy, constant need for bathrooms, numerous doctors' appointments, and frequent hospitalizations.

I had given up the presidency of the ostomy organization to encourage the growth of new leadership. I no longer had an ostomy and didn't want to lie about it. However, I also did not want to suggest to people that they should have it "put back." I had done far better with the ostomy even in its primitive days.

Soon I became involved in the National Foundation of Ileitis and Colitis (now the Crohn's & Colitis Foundation of America). The Detroit group was just starting. We met in each other's homes and started to build our dreams for the future. Many of these dreams are now fulfilled.

I became program vice-president and was leading many of the meetings. Frequently, people would come up to me after the meeting and ask for advice. I even started getting calls from others who were having difficulty living with IBD. Often I felt that I was doing therapy without a license. I toyed with the idea of going back to school, but it seemed formidable. Larry, too, had thought of returning to school and had become interested in a psychology program. He started classes immediately. It took me a semester to gather the courage to try.

I had heard of a marriage counseling program at the University of Detroit. The program was highly regarded, but equally important to me was the convenient parking. All the classes and the clinic were then held in one building. It seemed like something I could handle.

Just filling out all the application forms seemed overwhelming. I saw a counselor and was told that I would need some prerequisites before I was even eligible for the program. At first, I took just one class. Then I took two. Later I was able to handle a full program. One day I looked around the classroom and realized that my fellow students were young enough to be my children, but I was so excited to be in school again that that was hardly a concern.

My health seemed to be holding up, and I managed the first year. However, at the end of that year, I was taking final exams when I noticed I was bleeding. I called Dr. Feld, and he said "Cross your fingers, and cross your legs, and if it doesn't stop by tomorrow, come in." I took my final but then had to see him the next day. He suspected cancer and recommended some testing and then possibly a hysterectomy.

For the second time I thought that my life might be over. I remember walking around taking in the beauties of nature and being even more sensitive to the love around me.

Everything in life seems to have a purpose. This period was no exception. We had become friendly with Harold Ogust who ran the "Travel with Goren" Bridge cruises which Larry and I had taken from time to time. Harold had just been diagnosed with cancer and would not see anybody. But I knew that he couldn't refuse to see me now. I didn't want to wait until there was a definite diagnosis. If I did have cancer, I was afraid I wouldn't be able to travel later. So Larry and I went off to New York to see Harold and his wife Jean.

The tests came back, positive. I was scheduled to have a hysterectomy. Fortunately, it was now summer vacation, and I wouldn't miss any classes. After the hysterectomy Dr. Feld was pretty sure that they had removed all the cancer. Larry and I had planned a trip to France, and we set off. I saw the Louvre in a wheel chair, but by then that seemed to be an advantage rather than a disadvantage.

There was a new problem, however. While I had been in the hospital for the hysterectomy, doctors found that I had a kidney stone. They wanted to operate again. I promised that when I returned from France I would take care of this, and I did. My travel schedule ended with a trip to the operating room.

Next on my agenda was getting accepted into the actual marriage counseling program at the University of Detroit. Fifteen candidates were admitted each year, and many more applied. I was concerned that I would be rejected because I had a serious illness and had spent so much time in the hospital. Yet I didn't want to lie. What I did do is turn how I had handled this illness into a convincing argument for my acceptance. This approach has served me well.

I can't describe the excitement I felt when I learned that I had been admitted to the program. The next two years flew by. I had thought that I already knew a lot about psychology, but the new information seemed endless. If a professor digressed, it didn't matter to me. Everything was fascinating. One day as I was intent on recording every word, I felt a gentle nudge. The student next to me was saying, "You don't have to take that down, Audrey. It won't be on the test." She didn't realize that my goals were much more than having answers for a test.

During our group therapy course we were encouraged to conduct our own group. I was anxious to start a group for ileitis and colitis patients. I asked Dr. Dick Spain, our group therapy teacher, to be my co-therapist. He was delighted to have a ready-made group, and I was happy to have someone with experience as a co-therapist.

The first group was very successful, and more followed. My husband, now working on his doctorate in psychology, joined me as a co-therapist for a couples group dealing with IBD. We were all thrilled with what was happening, and Dick suggested we submit our work for presentation. The International Group Psychotherapy Association accepted our paper, and we were off to Copenhagen, Denmark, to present it. That was the beginning of numerous presentations. The first was especially exciting because I was still just a student and already involved in something that was so important to me.

Still, there were short trips to the hospital that necessitated calling patients to reschedule their appointments. But in May of 1979, I graduated. This time I marched in the procession and made it across the stage with ease. My family cheered, although my daughter Karen said that she loved it when they called my name but found the rest rather boring. Boring it was, but there was no way I was going to miss *this* graduation.

Now I was ready to find a job. I had been doing my internship at a Ford Hospital satellite in Dearborn, Michigan. I was seeing a few patients there, and after I graduated I was paid to continue seeing them. I was so excited about my first pay check that I wanted to frame it. I had never believed that I could hold a job.

Ford required a physical examination before they would hire me. I was honest about my medical history. Shortly after, I was told that my physical condition would prevent me from being hired. I was ready to take it to court, but the department head backed down and said they just weren't hiring at that time.

Meanwhile, Larry was completing his Ph.D. internship at Sinai Hospital. One day, while walking through the halls, he stopped to admire the decor in a psychiatrist's office. They talked for awhile. Keith Lepard told him that he was a surgeon and was now finishing a psychiatric residency. He mentioned he was interested in working with individuals with ostomies. Larry explained that his wife was also interested in therapy with individuals dealing with all aspects of IBD. Ironically, Keith had been a surgical resident when I was in the hospital with my first ostomy. I had told him about the ostomy organization, and now our paths were crossing again.

A few weeks later, Keith and I arranged to have lunch. We became excited about the possibility of working together. However, we both were looking for employment and left it at that.

At that time, I was putting together my 12-week group therapy program for individuals with ileitis and colitis. I had called it "A Bridge to Therapy." My good friend Edie Broida labored over it with me until we had the program perfected.

Then I received a call from Keith Lepard. He had recently interviewed at Medical Center Psychiatric Associates in the Detroit Medical Center. He had told them about me, and they were interested in my work.

So with my group program in hand, I went to the interview at MCPA. My idea at the time was to take this program to all the hospitals, but the psychiatrists there thought it would make more sense to work from one central place. I left the office and went home. I told Larry, "I think I have a job, but I'm not sure."

Yes, I did have a job. I had never thought that I would be able to work, and now I had an office of my own and my name on the door and I would be paid for what I enjoyed doing!

The day they put my name on the door, I beamed. I was finally a career woman. As I was about to go in to see a client, the chief psychiatrist, Dr. Robert Niccolini, asked if I was having problems at home. I wasn't sure what he was talking about, but I had to go into session. As soon as I finished, I asked what he meant. He said, "You know we use the telephone lines for emergency calls, and we can't have your children tying up the phones." I still wasn't sure what was going on so I called home.

Karen, who was eight at the time, answered the phone. "Did you call the office?" I asked. She said that she had, but she was upset because the lady was "playing games" with her and wouldn't let her talk to me. Karen had been connected to the taped message and wasn't aware that it wasn't a real person. I asked her what she did then.

"Oh," said Karen, "since she was playing a game, Bob and I decided to play a game."

"What game did you play?" I asked nervously.

"Oh, we just sang her a song."

"And what song was that?" I asked with growing apprehension.

"Oh, just something we learned on the playground. Ta rah rah boom te aye; how did you get that way?" She then continued the long detailed song.

"You are never to call the office again, unless it is an emergency!" I admonished. This was not a great beginning to my becoming a career woman.

From that point on, however, my career moved swiftly ahead. I presented my work frequently and fulfilled the requirements for becoming a marriage counselor, a fellow and diplomate of the American Board of Medical Psychotherapists, and a full member of both the American Group Psychotherapy Association and the American Marriage and Family Association. I was asked to be on the Hutzel Hospital Staff in Detroit, and Larry and I started the Center for Coping with Chronic Illness.

At the Foundation for Ileitis and Colitis (CCFA) I had become the psychological liaison. In that capacity I originated the "Coping Conference."

The first conference was held in 1981 at Hutzel Hospital. Fewer than

40 people attended. Those that did, however, were very enthusiastic.

Now the coping conference has become a program that is repeated here in Michigan every year. Each year we alternate having it in the Detroit Metropolitan area and in the outlying communities. We now have to limit attendance to one hundred people. Many individuals have benefitted from attending these conferences, which are duplicated around the country.

Serving on the board for the CCFA led to my writing the "Ask Audrey" column. This book will offer these columns to a wider audience.

Until 1984 my health remained fairly stable. I was used to the limitations of the illness and had found ways of getting around them. However, in 1984 my current internist, Dr. Sheldon Kantor, became disturbed that my ileum was starting to close at the point of the anastomosis (where they had connected the last surgery). He felt he had done what he could and suggested that I consult the Cleveland Clinic.

So in 1984, in addition to planning for moving both my office and home, my son's confirmation, my daughter's bat mitzvah, the banquet for our class reunion and a shower for my sister-in-law, I went to Cleveland for my second ileostomy.

In many ways it was easier than the first. For one thing, appliances had improved, and the health care providers were more knowledgeable. But it was still difficult being away from my support system. I was very touched by the friends and family who drove to Cleveland to be with me. The doctors again found kidney stones and wanted to operate. They were also afraid that I didn't have enough bowel left to receive adequate nutrition. The doctors wanted me to start TPN (total parenteral nutrition) and take care of the kidney stone as soon as possible. I was anxious to return home, and at that time TPN or another operation seemed overwhelming.

During this difficult period I had been working with Dr. Jason Bodzin on the CCFA board. He had been involved with the coping conferences. He could see that I just didn't look healthy and suggested TPN. I was concerned that it would make me an invalid, and we discussed this at length. Finally I agreed to have a port inserted and we started a process for which I am so grateful today. (See article "A Psychologist Copes.") The kidney stones were later dissolved by lithotripsy, another new procedure. Twice, I was admitted to the hospital for lithotripsy, but this required just a few days, not like the many weeks of recuperating from surgery in the past.

In the past few years I've had a few TPN port infections that required hospitalization, even though Larry and I are extremely careful. Being in the hospital those times was especially frustrating when there was so much to do. One time I received permission to leave the hospital for a few hours so that I could go back to the office to conduct my group therapy sessions.

In recent years I've been fortunate and I enjoy good health. I can do simple activities that I used to feel were impossible. I savor each day. I know that I have no guarantees with a chronic illness. I also realize that nobody else has a guarantee of good health either. They just think they do.

It's been a long journey for me and I've learned much along the way. I have had the advantage of having a wonderful support system. Larry has always been an active participant in my quest for health. My family and friends have been very special. However, I have learned that living a good life and enjoying supportive friends and family requires effort. In the various "Ask Audrey" columns, I've tried to share with you what I've learned both personally and professionally.

Putting this book together has taken much more time than I anticipated. However, if life is just a little easier for even one IBD patient, then it all will have been worthwhile. Years ago, in one of our groups at the Center for Coping with Chronic Illness, a young man with IBD said, "Before I came here, I felt that my illness was taking me for a ride. Now I feel like I'm the driver and the illness is just a passenger." After you read this book, you, too, may be a driver.

PART II:
A PSYCHOLOGIST
COPES

The following article was reprinted from "Caring for People," a publication of Caremark, Inc, Summer, 1989.

EDITOR'S NOTE: As a medical psychotherapist on the staff at Hutzel Hospital in Detroit and as director of the Center for Coping with Chronic Illness, Audrey Kron works with patients and family members affected by chronic illness.

Married, with three children, Audrey lives in a suburb of Detroit, and has coped with the ups and downs of Crohn's disease (a chronic inflammatory disease of the intestinal tract) for more than 30 years.

Audrey is an active volunteer with the Michigan chapter of the National Foundation for Ileitis and Colitis, and she serves as the NFIC's psychological liaison: writing a column, conducting the coping conference, and helping with the visiting program. She was recently honored with the Humanitarian of the Year award by the Michigan NFIC.

Audrey, who enjoys traveling, had just returned from a trip to India, Africa, and Israel when she took time out to talk about "coping" with *Caring for People*.

• • • • • • • • • • •

As told to Lakshmi Menon:

"Cinderella," I used to call myself. If I didn't get home by a certain time most nights, I couldn't make it to work the next morning. Because I am on total parenteral nutrition (TPN), I have to be hooked up to a TPN pump so that the nourishment my body needs

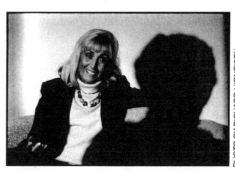

"Cultivate your sense of humor. It will make you feel better and put others at ease with your condition."

PHOTO BY RICHARD HIRNEISEN

can be pumped directly into my system. I am hooked up to the pump for 14 hours three nights a week and at least seven hours three other nights. Thus, when I began treatment, my pump and I often stayed home.

I guess I've come a long way since then. I was out on the dance floor the other night and a lady said to me, "You don't have to carry your purse with you while you're dancing; no one will take it." She was looking at the bag slung over my shoulder. What she didn't realize was that it held my portable pump—feeding me while I enjoyed the evening out. The point is, with a little planning, I can

ASK AUDREY

21

now pretty much go anywhere I want. As I become more experienced, I find I'm less fearful and more determined to enjoy myself and be thankful for the good times.

I can't say it has always been this way. I've had Crohn's disease since I was 16 years old, and I've had an ileostomy since 1984. The surgery was difficult and starting TPN was overwhelming. But we all get discouraged at some time or other. Coping is a question of finding the right tools to deal with every new situation. I was fortunate to have Dr. Jason Bodzin at Mt. Carmel Hospital in Detroit and the wonderful people at Caremark's Detroit branch guiding me through the new experience of being on TPN. Proper education is an important part of coping.

I don't go around thinking, "Why me?" Nobody gets through life without having to deal with something, and Crohn's disease happens to be what I have to handle. So, instead, I count my blessings. It's sort of like being on a diet: The best approach is to think about what you can eat, rather than focusing on what you can't. With illness, it's what you have now, not what's been taken away, that counts.

A good support system is a tremendous source of strength when you are feeling down. When you are young and ill, you sometimes worry that no one will want you. When my husband married me, he knew I was sick. It takes a special person to marry you and want to be with you when you aren't feeling well. In a sense, an illness can sometimes help separate out people who would leave you when times are bad.

You have to be able to discuss your fears and limitations with those close to you, but it's important not to turn your support system into a "give-me," one-way relationship. Becoming involved with others and shifting your focus away from yourself is one good way to avoid depression. I try to do things for others during the times that I feel good. I've found that if you are concerned about others, they are willing to be concerned about you.

Cultivating interests, reading, and becoming involved in activities can take your mind off your problems. For example, I do a lot of community service work. When I used to be in the hospital frequently, I took up duplicate bridge. I'm a terrible bridge player, and it took all my mental energy to think of what cards to play, so I couldn't think about the pain at the same time. My work as a psychotherapist has been especially rewarding. It keeps me involved with people and ideas, and it has helped me understand myself better. My son Michael once said to me, "Mom, you've certainly put your illness to good use."

It's also helpful to have a sense of humor about things. The TPN pump that I used to have was rather cumbersome. We had it on rollers, and it looked something like a vacuum cleaner. Though I couldn't get it into a car, I could take it around on short walks and in elevators. So when we travelled, I'd put a scarf around it to match my outfit and take it down to the hotel restaurant for dinner, and everyone thought I was vacuuming the carpet!

Time management, energy management, and stress management: These are the keys to keeping my illness from overwhelming me. If I can keep control over these areas, I control the way I live, and that helps me get the most out of life.

A lot of time is taken just treating my disease, so I've learned to prioritize—to decide what's worth spending time on, and what's not. And I've learned to use my energy in the best way possible so that I don't tire myself out unnecessarily. Before I go somewhere, I'll phone to make sure they have what I want. In the kitchen, I sit down on a stool while I work. I also have a little camp stool that I can carry around like a purse. So if I have to wait in line at the grocery store, I can just open it up and sit.

Planning ahead is one way to avoid stress. The boys are now 28 and 21, and my daughter is 17, but when they were little, I was in the hospital so much that I had to make sure the house could run without me. I used to have menus typed up so that whoever was coming to take care of the kids knew what they would eat. When we would go out to dinner or travel, we'd call ahead and ask to make any necessary arrangements. Soon, I'll be going to my daughter's school play. I've already made sure that I will have an aisle seat, so if I need to leave to use the ladies' room, I can do it without disturbing anyone.

It's important to put things in perspective. I think we sometimes get ourselves over-burdened because we can't say "no" or because we can't delegate jobs to others. But you find that things do get attended to, even if you're not around. It may not be quite the way you would do it, but what needs to be done gets done. Whenever things didn't go exactly right, my son used to say, "It's not the end of the world, Mom." I find he is right. What seems like such a crisis at the moment is something I'm not going to care about a short time later.

ASK AUDREY

Naturally, I don't want to suffer any more than I have to, so I try to make my situation as comfortable as possible. In hospitals, I decorate my room, and bring the things I want to have around me. If a procedure is painful, I try to concentrate on something else. When a needle is being put in, I take a deep breath and take myself away to a peaceful place, with the sun shining and flowers blooming—some place soothing and comforting.

Taking time out for relaxing and playing is also important. I make sure that I don't have to go to the hospital to get the rest I need. I like to read or just be with friends or family. There's nothing wrong with pampering yourself once in a while: It makes you feel good and that's a legitimate goal.

Doing things by myself, for myself, helps me feel that I'm in control of my illness. I used to be very dependent. I never thought that I'd be able to work. Going back to school, when my youngest child was in kindergarten, was frightening. But I started with one course, then two, and gradually worked up to a full load.

The more you do things for yourself, the better you feel. For example, do little things like keeping a pitcher of water beside you instead of having to ask someone every time you need a drink.

I find I do well when I set goals for myself. Short-term goals help me get through the day. My current short-term goal is to learn to use the computer. My long-term goal is to write a book about my experiences. My goals change as I change. Right now, I have a short-term goal of unpacking and getting my laundry done after my most recent trip!

And when something seems insurmountable, I break it up into parts. I tell myself, today I'll work on this for 20 minutes, and, when I do, it's better than feeling frustrated by not doing it at all. The idea of cleaning my house may be overwhelming, but if I decide to do just one table today, and then I do it, I feel more positive about the whole thing.

The whole point, I think, whether you are ill or not, is to develop a sense of purpose. I want to help people cope with chronic illness, and knowing that I'm doing that helps me immensely. Knowing that there's more of that work to be done, and that there's so much in life that I still want to do—those are the things that keep me going. ◆

PART III:
GENERAL INFORMATION ABOUT CHRONIC ILLNESS

Dear Audrey,

I am 13 years old, and my parents told me that my colitis is a chronic disease. I know what a terminal disease is. Does chronic mean the same thing? I'm too frightened and embarrassed to ask my parents or my doctor. Please just answer me in your column. —W.S.

Dear W.S.,

There are two issues to address in your letter. First is not being able to talk to your parents or doctor, and the second is the meaning of "chronic" illness.

As far as talking to your parents or doctor is concerned, it can make matters much easier if they know what your fears or misconceptions are. They certainly can give you the facts that you need to understand your illness. In addition, just talking about your fears is often helpful. If for some reason at this time you don't feel comfortable talking with either your parents or your doctor, try and find someone that you can talk to. It might be a teacher, counselor, member of the clergy, parent of a friend, etc. Also, don't forget that your local Crohn's and Colitis Foundation of America chapter has literature on every aspect of IBD. There may even be support groups available to you.

The meaning and acceptance of "chronic illness" are issues with which many individuals with IBD struggle. We know that IBD is not a terminal illness. A terminal illness is an illness that results in death. "Chronic," on the other hand, means that the illness is always there, but the symptoms are not expected to cause one to die.

Chronic is also different from acute. An acute medical problem can be a broken leg, flu, or anything that has a definite short-term beginning and end. Though a chronic illness is always with you, the symptoms aren't. During some periods one can feel as if nothing is wrong, and, at other times, one can be seriously ill.

Some individuals stay at one stage of the illness all the time, but this is less common. It's like a roller coaster ride. At first, it may seem completely out of control. However, gradually learning more about the illness, though not totally eliminating the difficult stages, makes those times easier to manage. Sometimes preventative steps can be taken to lessen the symptoms.

Many people talk of the "time bomb" effect, the feeling of not knowing when "it" will strike. But one can be prepared for bombs, and one can be prepared for a recurrence of the IBD. First, it is important to do everything necessary to postpone the recurrence. We do not know the cause of these illnesses so we don't know for sure what would prevent them. But we do know some factors that may help control the disease. Talk to your doctor about medication. Make sure that your body is getting the nutrition and rest that it needs so that you are not vulnerable. And reduce stressful situations in your life. We don't believe that stress causes the illness, but we do know that stress often makes an existing illness worse.

We haven't yet found a cure for these diseases; they can still recur even with excellent care. Learning to live with the uncertainty requires great skill. Because there is no schedule for a chronic illness, how you feel may vary from week to week, day to day or even hour to hour. Others may have difficulty understanding the shifts in your health. It makes it much easier if you educate your teachers and friends. There are very helpful booklets for teachers available at the CCFA office. You can give your friends literature on IBD, bring them to a CCFA meeting or just tell them about the illness in a brief way.

It is also necessary to plan your time wisely. Utilize the periods when the illness is in remission to prepare for times when you aren't feeling as well. Squirrels gather their nuts for the winter. You can learn from them. This may mean taking care of activities that require more energy while you are able to do so. You can also have projects planned for when you aren't feeling your best. It might be an easy reading book, a comic tape, or some music you wanted to hear. Having what you need near your bed can come in handy for the days when moving around is difficult.

Being prepared is a highly individual matter. Everyone has different needs.

ASK AUDREY

It's important that you know your needs so that you can better tend to them during difficult times.

You can have a chronic illness and rarely be bothered by it. I sincerely hope that yours will be like that. Since we just don't know when the disease might reappear, it's better to be prepared, and then be pleasantly surprised if these preparations prove to be unnecessary. Good luck, and don't hesitate to write if you have any other questions.

Notes

PART IV:
PRACTICAL
SUGGESTIONS

Dear Audrey,
   My diarrhea is so bad that I've become completely housebound. I'm frightened to go any place. How do others manage?   —G.R.

Dear G.R.,
   Needing a bathroom at a moment's notice can really cause anxiety. It's often tempting to just stay home where you can feel secure. However, my experience has been that most people feel much better when they can get out of the house and partake in a somewhat normal social life. My column of January 1984 addresses that issue. I'm going to repeat it with several additions:

Q "I was recently diagnosed as having Crohn's disease. I have constant diarrhea, and I'm afraid to go to most places for fear of having an accident or being embarrassed because I have to go so frequently. Is this illness going to stop my social life? —B.E.

A I can appreciate how concerned you are at the moment. Most individuals with IBD are able to enjoy their social life once they learn how to handle their illness. Talking about accidents is very difficult. But I have found that once you can talk about this problem, it is easier to solve. I am always amazed by the inventive solutions that others have developed. Here are some suggestions that have proven helpful. (We hope that our readers will share their tips with us, too. Remember that the illness varies not only from individual to individual but also in different ways for the same individual).

• Consult your doctor. There may be some medication that will reduce the diarrhea. Remember that different medications work at different times for the same individual.

- Observe your diet and learn which foods cause more diarrhea for you. Foods and drinks usually fall into three categories. First, there are those that are always safe. Second, there are those that sometimes are OK and sometimes cause trouble. Lastly, there are those that always give you trouble. Stick with the first group for important occasions and do your experimenting at a time when you'll be home.

- Plan ahead. Know where lavatories are located before you have to use them.

- Learn the obvious places to stop. You can't go far today without a fast food restaurant. McDonald's even puts out lists of their locations. In regular restaurants, walk in with authority and either head for the rest room or ask where it's located. Nobody knows if you are staying for a meal or not. If you feel uncomfortable about using the rest room and not eating there, just order a cold drink or something to go.

- Map out emergency stops along the paths that you travel. There are probably many rest rooms that are open to the public. Have you tried office buildings, shopping centers, hospitals, large retail stores, gas stations? It's important that you check them out ahead of time. When you are in a hurry, there's no time to negotiate for keys.

Now let's deal with rest rooms that are closed to the public. Supermarkets, small retail stores, banks, etc., all have rest rooms for their employees. Often you will be told that they don't have a rest room or that you can't use it. Again, it's difficult to negotiate when you are in an emergency situation. However, it is often possible to phone ahead of time, to tell the manager that you have IBD and frequently need to use a bathroom at a moment's notice. You can even give them some literature from CCFA. Sometimes that will be enough. However, if they are still reluctant, you can say that you need bathroom privileges to patronize their business. If they still say "no," then take your business elsewhere. If they agree, get it in writing.

There may be someone else in charge when you hurriedly rush to the rest room!

When traveling, you can use gas stations and rest stops. However, restaurants, motels and hotels are usually much nicer. You can even obtain a catalogue of Holiday Inns along the way to know exactly where they are. If you are leaving the country, make sure you know how to ask, "Where is the bathroom?" in the native language.

For entertainment events, arrange for an aisle seat. Ask the usher what time the intermission begins. This will enable you to make a fast exit just before it starts and avoid the long lines. It's also helpful if you know the layout of the auditorium, so that you are not at the opposite side of the rest rooms. You can usually obtain this information when you are purchasing tickets.

With some teachers or employers it is helpful to explain ahead of time that there may be times when you have to leave quickly. Remember the way you tell them is very important. Here, too, some CCFA literature from our School Awareness Committee is helpful.

Some individuals with IBD believe it would be helpful to have a card that would explain the situation and perhaps make it easier to get into any bathrooms. The foundation is working on this. If you think this is a good idea, drop them a note. If you want to work on the committee, let them know.

- Work on any emotional concerns that you have. We don't believe the disease is caused by emotions, but sometimes emotions can play a part in increasing the diarrhea. Even individuals without IBD are often affected physically when under stress.

- Most of all, remember that you are much more conscious of what is going on than are others. Keep a smile on your face and try not to feel embarrassed. You are doing the best you can in a difficult situation, and you should be proud that you are able to deal with it.

<u>Notes</u>

Dear Audrey,
How do you choose a doctor? I know it's an important decision, but I just don't know where to begin. —D.P.

Dear D.P.,
Choosing a doctor is very much like choosing a spouse. One person is not right for everyone. There are several steps you might take to ensure that you get the doctor that is best for you. They are as follows:

- Determine what kind of doctor you need. Nowadays, with specialization, someone with IBD might need a variety of doctors such as:

    An internist - for general health needs.

    A gastroenterologist - specifically for the IBD.

    A surgeon - if surgery is considered.

    A urologist - for matters concerning kidneys, prostate.

    A gynecologist - for childbirth or female problems.

    A rheumatologist - if there is any arthritis.

    An ophthalmologist - for any eye conditions.

    A dermatologist - for skin complications.

    A radiologist - for various x-rays.

    A psychologist - to help you cope more effectively.

- Once you have determined what kind of doctor is required, the next step is finding him or her. Some of the actions you can take are:

    Ask a doctor you already have and trust for recommendations.

    Ask your friends and family.

    Ask people at CCFA. Usually they have some recommendations for gastroenterologists, surgeons and other physicians.

Call your local medical society.

Call the hospital you would like to go to and ask for a referral.

- Now arrange for an interview (be willing to pay) or see if you can talk to the doctors or their receptionists for a few minutes on the phone. Prepare a list of questions to ask them. Some questions you might consider are:

  What are their credentials? Are they licensed? Where did they get their training? What is their specialty?

  What hospitals are they affiliated with?

  What are their office hours and how do they handle the time that they are not in the office?

  How do you reach them in an emergency?

  What are their fees?

  What insurance do they accept?

  Do they believe in sharing the information with you and consulting you on the decision, or do they consider all the facts and make what they consider the best decision? Which style do you want?

  Do you feel comfortable talking to them? Do they pay attention to you while you are talking, or do they seem preoccupied?

  How comfortable are they in working with your other doctors or in making referrals when necessary?

Is their office staff helpful? Are you able to get your questions answered and get to the doctor when it's important?

How long do you have to wait for an appointment?

A gastroenterologist specializes in IBD, but how much experience have the other doctors had with colitis and Crohn's disease?

You can add other questions that seem appropriate for you. Remember to have your questions in front of you in writing. Jot down the answers as the doctor or their staff talk, or use a tape recorder. This may seem like a lot of work and may not be necessary for doctors you won't be seeing frequently. However, doctors such as your gastroenterologist are going to be with you for your lifetime. You don't want to have to choose someone when you're too sick to think clearly. Having a doctor that you can trust and work with is clearly worth this effort.

<u>Notes</u>

Dear Audrey,

I have colitis. My doctor says that I may have to be hospitalized in the near future. I have never been in the hospital and I am a little apprehensive. Do you have any tips to make my hospital stay easier?

—H.V.

Dear H.V.,

I can understand your apprehension. A hospital can be a formidable place for someone unfamiliar with hospital routine. Most of us, during the course of our lives, will have to spend some time in the hospital. The trick is to make your visit as comfortable for yourself as you can. The following tips may help you.

WHAT TO BRING:

- Nightclothes, slippers, robe, toiletries, and clothing for the trip home. When selecting nightclothes and robes, remember there may be times when you need to have I.V.'s. It is easier to get in and out of clothes that open all the way down or that you can step into.

  Of course, there may be times you will be required to wear the infamous "hospital gown." These gowns are notorious for not quite covering you. The problem is easily solved. For women: bring a long lovely ribbon. For men: a belt, wrapped around the waist, helps keep the gown closed. Another way to keep off the draft when those hospital gowns are imposed on you is to ask for two: put one on properly and the other on backward.

- A cardigan sweater makes a nice bed jacket if the room is too cold.

- A tape recorder. This can serve a multitude of purposes. Pre-tape your favorite music or comedy album, or borrow "talking books" from your local library (sometimes it is easier to listen than to read). Your family and friends can also tape messages for you to play when you are alone. Another important use for the tape recorder is having a record of the doctors' instructions. Ask your doctors for permission and then record what they have to say. Often when you see them, you don't absorb everything they relate, so it is helpful if you can replay the discussion (instructions) later.

• Scotch tape and some of your favorite pictures of family, friends, pets, or even soothing scenes that delight you. Most hospitals have some provision for patients to hang their get-well cards and photos. You can make your room cheerful and comforting.

• Magazines or books that you are in the middle of reading. It is often difficult to start a new book in the hospital. There are many interruptions in your reading time, and most people find that they need to read one level lower than they usually do. For instance, if you normally read serious literature, your might try a light novel.

• Pen and paper. You'll want to jot down questions for the doctors and nurses. You may want to list personal items you want brought from home or information you want to share with your family. It is a good idea to keep records of what's happening, such as symptoms, test results, and the medications you are receiving (when and how you are to get them). You may also want to keep records of some of the feelings you are having (this can be very therapeutic).

• Your personal phone book, stamps, and note paper.

• At least one day's supply of your medicines. It might take that long until your doctor's orders are received. You may also want to show your medications to the attending physician. This will answer some of the residents' questions regarding your medicines.

• Most important, a good attitude. Try to understand the viewpoint of all the people with whom you will come in contact in the hospital.

IN THE HOSPITAL:
• Adjust to the hospital schedule. This usually entails setting your watch ahead about two hours, as everything starts much earlier. It is almost

impossible to sleep in the busy hours of the morning. You are much better off getting up and ready early. At night, you will be more tired and can go to sleep earlier.

• Learn how everything in the room works. There are buttons to call the nurse, to raise and lower your bed, and to put out the light. Ask how they work. Often hospitals have a patient education booklet available. READ IT!

• Hospital food can be very bland. You may not even be able to have salt. Check with your doctor if you are allowed to have seasonings like Dash, garlic powder, tarragon, basil, dill, etc. If so, bring them with you to season your food. Sometimes this "spice of life" can make the hospital food taste more like home cooking. You will get a daily menu. On this menu you're usually able to write in simple items that aren't listed (like a tuna sandwich—if you are allowed to eat it). Call for the dietitian and work out a food plan that works best for you.

• Learn the duties of the various people on the health care team. During the day just some of the people you may encounter are doctors, nurses, aides, volunteers, students, housekeepers, x-ray technicians and dieticians. It's wise to ask their names and know their roles. For example, don't ask the nurse when you are going home. It is the doctor who makes that final decision. However, if you need to know something about your daily routine, then you'd better ask the nurse. Everyone plays a unique part in your recovery.

• Know the medicines prescribed for you. Know how you are to receive these medicines—orally, intravenously, or by injection. Write it down so you don't forget, as they can change from day to day.

• Know what diagnostic procedures are being done. Ask to have them explained. For some tests, a mild sedative will make the procedure much easier. If you don't ask, you won't know. Take along a magazine or something to hold your interest when you go for the tests. Sometimes you have to wait in the hallway, and a pleasant distraction makes the time pass a little faster.

• Be assertive: Unless you ask, you cannot expect to have your needs met. Find out if your hospital has patient representatives or coordinators. They can be very helpful in assisting you with any problems you may have regarding your hospitalization.

• Don't hesitate to ask for the professional that meets your needs. Hospitals employ social workers, dietitians, psychologists and physical therapists, to name a few. Utilize them.

• Ask for and get explanations from doctors, nurses and technicians about procedures you are to undergo. Ask about your records, x-rays, etc. It is important to have access to them for future reference. Become a partner with the health care professionals in your health care.

Hospitalization does not have to be frightening! It is up to you. The key is thoughtful preparation.

Notes

Dear Audrey,

I feel that I cope quite well with my Crohn's Disease, but I'm still having difficulty dealing with the pain. Any suggestions would be most welcome.

—N.B.

Dear N.B.

Pain is often the body's way of alerting us. We can consider pain our friend in warning us that something needs attention. There are some people that don't experience pain, and it make life very dangerous because they don't receive important signals.

The first step you can take, once the pain signals you, is to contact your doctor and make sure that immediate attention isn't required.

If the pain is severe, the doctor will consider medication or even surgery. Or your doctor may suggest T.P.N. (total parenteral nutrition) to rest the bowel or perhaps a more restricted or liquid diet.

Learn to be able to describe your pain. Is it crampy or sharp? Is it constant or is it worse after eating? Do you also have a fever or diarrhea? It is important to be able to give your doctor as much information as possible.

What I want to address now is how to handle the pain when your doctor has done all that is indicated.

It's helpful to remember that the mind has difficulty thinking of more than one item at a time. The pain always feels worse in the middle of the night when that is all you are concentrating on. So one obvious solution is to keep your mind busy. Of course, this isn't always easy when you are in pain. When you are feeling well, you might want to prepare some audio or video tapes that will hold your interest when you need to divert your thoughts. Calling a good friend or even somebody that needs your help might also work for you.

Something else to be aware of is that the body tenses up when there is pain. Then the tension causes more pain. To break this cycle, you might try some relaxation exercises. Again, you should be prepared ahead of time with those exercises. The library and bookstores are filled with books on various forms of relaxation such as TM, yoga, and visualization. Find one that works for you. You can also alleviate pain sometimes by just taking a hot bath or having a loved one give you a massage. Know that most pain is time limited. Remember that "this too shall pass."

Try to understand the pain. Is it telling you something about your emotional life? For example, if the pain occurs every time you visit your mother-in-law, it would help to work out your feelings about this relationship. IBD is not believed to be caused by stress, but sometimes stress can exacerbate the illness. If you can figure out what is causing your stress, it may prove helpful.

Your pain could also be telling you something else. Did you overtire yourself, or perhaps eat something that disagreed with you? A journal may help you to identify any patterns in the pain. If you can pinpoint it in any way, it makes it easier to overcome.

Sometimes there doesn't seem to be anything that can be done to alleviate the pain. In most cases your doctor will allow you to have some medication on hand for such an emergency. You do have to be careful, however, because narcotics may constipate you and cause more trouble if there is an obstruction, and addiction creates even more problems.

If the pain persists, consider a second opinion, just to make sure that there isn't anything else that can be done. Another alternative is reading books on coping with pain. One such book is *Free Yourself From Pain*, by Dr. David F. Bresler, Director of the UCLA Pain Control Unit.

During the course of this illness, most of us will experience pain from time to time. If we understand it, learn ways to ease it and keep our minds on the positive aspects of our lives, it will become bearable. With some practice it is possible to take ourselves away from the situation mentally. We have all heard of people who walk on hot coals or endure severe torture by using the power of their minds.

Finally, we can learn from pain the pleasure of not having pain. Experiencing pain helps us appreciate the wonders of life during our pain-free days.

<u>Notes</u>

Dear Audrey,
I have to have frequent blood tests and I.V.'s to keep my body chemistry at the proper levels. Unfortunately, I have veins that are not easy to find. I'm always frightened when I know that I have to have blood drawn. I worry about it for weeks before it happens. Is there anything you can suggest that might make it easier for me? **—B.T.**

Dear B.T.,
First of all, let's talk about the agony that you put yourself through prior to having your blood drawn. Often the fears are much worse than the reality. One reason many people fear something is that they feel they don't have any control over the situation. Let me make some suggestions that will help give you a sense of control.

• Get to know the blood and I.V. technicians by name. They are people, too, and respond better when treated with respect.

• Notice which ones seem to do better with you and arrange to have them either draw your blood or start your I.V. If necessary, talk to your doctor about requesting these particular individuals.

• In most circumstances, after three tries, ask for someone else. After technicians miss three times, they often become nervous and unable to accomplish the task.

• Sometimes warm compresses will bring veins up when it is difficult to find them.

• Attitude plays an important part. If you are nervous, it becomes harder to draw your blood or get into your veins. Try some visualization to relax yourself. Think about a favorite peaceful spot. Sometimes just visualizing the blood flowing or gushing can create a positive feeling that actually works.

- Do not abuse your veins by taking unnecessary tests. Keep a record of each time you take a blood test. Often one doctor can get the results from another and spare a precious vein. Sometimes microtests can be run so that less blood is necessary.

- Pay attention to what is happening and ask questions. Where is the best site for you? What kind of needle works best? Are your veins close to the surface? Do your veins collapse? Sometimes explaining what works best can give the person trying to get into your veins helpful clues.

- Don't be intimidated. You can be pleasant, but it's *your* body, and you have the ultimate responsibility for taking care of it.

- Make sure that you are not dehydrated before taking the blood test. It makes it more difficult. If the test doesn't prohibit it, try to drink some extra water beforehand.

- Give yourself a pep talk. Tell yourself, "I can handle the discomfort. It's for a limited time. It could be worse." Think of someone that has to endure something much more painful.

- Reward yourself. Think of your reward while they are drawing your blood. It doesn't have to be anything big, but just something that would be a treat: going to a special movie, getting a new book, lunching with a friend, allotting some time just for yourself, buying something frivolous!

With all of these hints, taking blood tests or getting I.V.'s should be much easier for you. If, however, you are still having problems, perhaps it would be helpful to talk to someone about it. A professional can help you to understand where your fears originate.

You may also have noticed that some of these hints can easily be applied to other unpleasant tests. All in all, you will find it much easier if you take control of the situation instead of worrying about it.

ASK AUDREY

50

<u>Notes</u>

Dear Audrey,

I have IBD and feel very anxious about traveling. I used to love to travel, but now I feel that my traveling days are over. Are others with IBD able to travel? If so, how do they manage it? I have so many concerns when I even think of taking a trip. —S.S.

Dear S.S.,

The answer to your question is, of course people with IBD travel! They travel all over the country and all over the world. What's important, though, is that, like boy scouts, they are prepared. Since you weren't specific about what it was that was concerning you, let me just give some general tips to alleviate anxiety when traveling.

• Have your doctor write a note that tells about your illness, your medications and any treatment that might be necessary in out-of-the-ordinary circumstances.

• Take all your medications with you. Know what medications you are taking, the strength and the frequency, so that you may relate that information to another doctor if necessary. It's wise to carry a written list in your wallet.

• Have your doctor recommend a doctor in the area or areas in which you will be traveling. You probably won't need to use this information, but it will make you feel more confident.

• Learn to budget your energy. When you are feeling your best, be careful not to tire yourself. Allow times to rest. When you are feeling "fair," learn to conserve your energy. Use a portable seat for times you might otherwise have to stand. When you feel weaker, consider using a wheelchair for long hauls. Many public places such as museums, zoos, etc., have wheelchairs available. This may be hard to accept, but remember it's only a temporary measure. If a wheelchair will enable you to travel with your family, consider it. Isn't it better than giving up your pleasure totally?

- Speaking of wheelchairs, remember that wheelchairs are available at airports. Call ahead and you can have one waiting and avoid the long walks to and from the airplane. Also, most airports have chauffeured electric carts available, if need be.

- *When you are flying*, tell the steward or stewardess if you have any concerns. They can be extremely considerate.

  Call ahead if you are on a special diet. The airlines can usually provide a special meal.

  Look at the layout of the plane and make sure that you request a seat near the bathroom. It's helpful to call ahead and explain your situation to be assured of an appropriate seat.

  If you're not feeling well, you can request permission to board ahead of time. That way you'll avoid the rush.

  Make sure you keep at least two to three days supply of medication in your carry-on bag, just in case your luggage is lost.

- *When you are traveling by car*, there are also special arrangements you can make. Pack a cooler with something to drink (avoid dehydration), a pillow and blanket (rest between destinations) and a guidebook for Holiday Inns, Best Western Motels, McDonald's or any franchise chain along the way that is apt to have clean bathrooms. You'll have the security of knowing that there's always a place to stop.

- If you're feeling really miserable, you might want to stay home. However, you can start planning your next trip.

- If you are going to a foreign country, try to learn at least a few key phrases in the native language. "Where's the bathroom?" is good for a start.

- Learning more about the place you are going can make the trip much more enjoyable. Many books are available in the travel section of your library.

- Above all, a positive attitude and a smile on your face will enhance the trip for you and the people you meet.

BON VOYAGE!

Notes

Dear Audrey,

I have Crohn's disease and have had a lot of surgery. Now my doctor is suggesting that I go on home TPN because I'm having a great deal of difficulty in absorbing my food. The mere thought of it terrifies me. Do you think I should consider this option? —E.B.

Dear E.B.,

Total parenteral nutrition (TPN) need not be a frightening proposition. It may even be a welcome addition to your life. However, there are many considerations. Because I'm not a doctor, I can't make the medical judgment for you. What I can do is offer information to guide your thinking process.

The first step is to determine if TPN is necessary in your particular case. Some of the questions you may ask are:

• What is the quality of your life now?

• Have you tried less dramatic measures such as food supplements?

• Did you seek a second opinion?

• Do you have confidence in your doctor?

• Does he or she consider TPN elective or essential?

If you should decide in favor of TPN, here are seven additional points to ponder.

1. Do you understand what home TPN is?
Very briefly, TPN is a method of feeding the necessary nutrients directly into the blood stream through an IV line. The term "home" just indicates that the recipient is taught how to continue this treatment at home. The more experience you have, the easier it will become.

2. Will you prefer the catheter to be outside the skin (a long-term silastic catheter often called a Hickman catheter) or an implanted port that is under the skin?

There are advantages and disadvantages to both. For example, the implanted port allows you to go swimming and take showers when the needle isn't in place. However, you do have to change the needle through the skin at least once a week.

3. Who will teach you how to manage the whole procedure? And, who is going to be your backup if you have difficulty?

There are several groups that provide this training and back-up-system in the home health care field. Choose your company carefully. It makes a major difference. Your training should start in the hospital.

4. How are you going to pay for the TPN?

TPN is very costly. Some insurance companies cover all or at least part of the charge. Medicaid also may be an alternative. Or you may have to use creativity to raise the money. Be sure you know your resources before you start.

5. Where are you going to store supplies?

Home TPN requires paraphernalia (such as syringes, sterile gloves, etc.). It helps if you use a linen closet, cupboard or some other place so that your home doesn't look like a hospital. Make sure it's an area away from pets and small children.

6. What is the quality of your support system?

TPN will affect your whole family. It's important that they be considered in this decision. A family member or friend should be trained as a back-up.

7. How is your emotional life at this time?

TPN will go much more smoothly if you take care of unsolved issues before you begin. Or, if this is not possible, at least tend to them while you are on TPN.

ASK AUDREY

When I started writing this column, I planned to show you ways that you could lead a fairly normal life on TPN. It may seem overwhelming to you, but planning can simplify the process. Once you have done the preliminary work, you will find that TPN can change your whole life for the better. The added nutrients will give you more strength than you have probably had for a long time. For example, if your body is low in vitamins or minerals they can just be added to the TPN solution.

There are many ways to make day-to-day life easier, to carry on important activities, and even to make all kinds of travel possible. I discuss these in other articles.

So, E.B., my advice is to not fear TPN. It is a wonderful way to deal with absorption problems. Your decision should be based on consideration of all aspects. Consult with your family and your doctor. Then come to an answer that is right for you. Good luck.

Notes

In a recent article I talked to E.B. about the decision to accept TPN (Total Parenteral Nutrition). At that time, I did promise that I would suggest ways to cope with TPN, once the decision has been made. So in this column I will deal with some helpful hints to make life on TPN easier. I will also answer some of the most frequently asked questions.

When I first heard about home TPN, it seemed that it would make me an invalid. Now, however, with increased knowledge and improvements in the field, I see TPN as an enrichment to life, not a detriment.

Like any other process, the more you learn about it the easier it becomes. The first coping skill is gaining information. Sit down with your doctor with a list of questions and have him or her explain the process in detail. The home health service that you deal with is also prepared to answer your questions and give you material to read. In addition, there is an organization for people on TPN. They will send you information free if you are on TPN. To reach them, write: Lifeline, Oley Foundation A-23, Albany Medical Center, Albany, N.Y. 12208.

Traveling need not be a problem. As many of you have heard me say before, it just requires advance planning. Portable machines that run on batteries are now available, so even visits to foreign countries pose no obstacle. Have a list of the supplies that you require. In some cases your home health service will even arrange to send them to you. Refrigeration is necessary for the TPN bags. Call ahead and make arrangements in the hotels where you are staying. For car trips you can use coolers with insulated bags and the plastic ice packs that can be frozen ahead of time.

Naturally, a portable IV stand is convenient away from home, but there is usually something around on which you can hang the TPN bag, such as a bedpost, chair, or a lamp. Be resourceful!

The whole process is easier if you develop a routine. It helps to put everything you need for each procedure in a basket or plastic bag. That way you won't be interrupted in the middle because you are missing something. It also serves as a check. If an item is left over, you know you overlooked a step.

POSTSCRIPTS
Here are some of the other frequently asked questions regarding TPN:

ASK AUDREY

- **Do I have to put the needle in every day?**
No. If you use the external catheter method, there is a permanent outlet, and no needle is required. If you have an implanted port, which is under the skin (generally in the chest or upper abdomen), the needle can stay in for a week.

- **Will having the needle hurt?**
Once the needle is in, you don't even feel it.

- **Will I have to have the infusion going all the time?**
This depends on your situation. Often schedules can be arranged so that you take it only while you are sleeping.

- **What happens in between infusions?**
You merely put a cap on the line (something you will be taught to do) and just tape it down. Women do have an advantage here since they can just tuck it into their bras.

- **Can I engage in sexual activities while the infusion is going?**
There is no reason to curtail your sexual life. In fact, the increased energy you will feel may enhance it.

- **Will I be tied down during the infusion?**
Complete mobility is possible. There are some pumps that are portable, and you can carry on regular daily activities while the IV is running.

- **Can I eat while I am on TPN?**
This depends on what the TPN is for. If you are using it to rest the bowel, your doctor may not want you to eat. If, however, it is to build you up, eating is usually permissible. You will not be as hungry, so the eating may be more recreational than a matter of necessity.

- **What are the biggest problems with TPN?**
The biggest problem is risk of infection. That's why it becomes imperative that you learn the proper techniques of administering the program.

- **Can I sleep while on TPN?**
Yes. The TPN is run through a pump that has alarm systems to wake you if something is wrong.

- **Do you have to stay on TPN forever?**
That depends on what determined the original choice of TPN. If it's to rest the bowel or just build you up, it may just be temporary. If it's for Short Bowel Syndrome it probably will be a longer-term therapy. However, in that case you may be able to cut down the amount of days you infuse as your nutrition improves.

- **Will life ever be normal again once I'm on TPN?**
At first, TPN may seem overwhelming, but you will be amazed at how quickly it can become just a routine part of your day.

- **Is it really worth the bother?**
Once on TPN, most people are thrilled with the results of getting the necessary nutrients into their system. The increased energy is a welcome relief.

Notes

Dear Audrey,

I have colitis, and my doctor told me that I might have to have an ostomy. I have been so upset since then that I haven't been able to think of anything else. I really don't know what to do. I'm writing to you in desperation. —D.S.

Dear D.S.

It's unfortunate that this idea has been so upsetting to you, but you certainly are not alone in your concerns. Most people with IBD worry, needlessly, about the possibility of having an ostomy. A lot of the concern comes from misinformation or lack of information. I don't know enough about your individual situation so I will deal with some of the more common concerns.

First, most people with IBD do not need ostomies. However, for some it is the treatment of choice. In the case of colitis, when it is indicated, an ostomy may be a cure.

Currently there are several alternative surgeries available. The rectal sparing endorectal pull-through has been very successful in colitis cases, especially with young people. If you want more information about alternative surgeries, contact a surgeon that has experience in this area.

However, it's not the choice of surgeries, or whether or not to have surgery, that bothers most people. It is often concerns connected with having an ostomy that are found most troublesome. One worry that arises is that there will be an unpleasant odor. That might have been true years ago. Now the appliances are odor-proof and leak-proof. You need only to learn how to apply them correctly. We are fortunate now to have the resources of many fine stoma therapists that are trained to help ostomates.

In addition to the concern about odor, you may fear that you will look different and have to wear special clothes. You *will* probably look different. You will probably look healthier! As far as clothes are concerned, you will find that you can wear just about everything you could before.

"Can I go swimming?" is another question many ask. It is all right to go swimming and also to engage in many other sports. In fact, you probably will be stronger and able to enjoy sports that were too tiring before.

The last concern, and one that often doesn't get asked, is "What about my sex life?" Or, if someone is unmarried, they may want to know, "Will

ASK AUDREY

anyone ever find me attractive?" Except in rare cases, ostomates enjoy a normal sex life. In fact, the new vitality often makes it better. The person that you want for a partner in life will see you as a whole person, not just an ostomate. Their concern will be that you are as healthy as you can be.

This is just a brief discussion about ostomies. An abundance of useful material is available. For additional information you can call the United Ostomy Association. Their number is 1-800-826-0826. My main concern is that you, D.S., and all my other readers do not fear having an ostomy. Chances are you won't need one, but even if it is necessary, it is nothing to dread. Roosevelt's quote, "There is nothing to fear but fear itself," certainly applies in this situation. The fear can drain you emotionally. If you still have concerns, talk to someone about them. Get some professional help. Don't just sit and worry.

Notes

PARTIV: PRACTICAL SUGGESTIONS

Dear Audrey,

I have had Crohn's disease for 12 years. I know that this may seem like a silly problem, but one of the hardest things for me to do is to get up in the morning. Is there anything that I can do that will help?

—L.E.

Dear L.E.

First of all, recognize that your problem is not silly. Many patients with IBD report the same feelings. When we're not feeling well, the simplest tasks seem overwhelming.

I have found that most of us feel better when we get up, wash, and comb our hair. Women feel better if they have their usual make-up on, and men if they shave. When you're not feeling well, it's easy to say "Why bother?" or "Who cares?" However, how we look often affects how we feel. Looking in the mirror at a disheveled person can only make you feel worse. When you look better, others respond to you in a more positive fashion.

I recognize that just getting up can be difficult, so we really have to motivate ourselves to take the first step. There are several ways to do this ourselves. One is having something special to look forward to do. It might be something appealing for breakfast, a favorite program you want to watch, a call to someone you like. It's not hard to find just one thing that would be rewarding.

Next, get as much ready as possible the day before. Sometimes just little things like picking out clothes, finding a belt, or looking for keys can make the whole process seem too much to handle if left for morning.

Have something planned to do each day. At all stages of the illness it is important to have some structure to the day. Be realistic about time. Allowing plenty of time for that extra trip to the bathroom avoids having to put additional stress on ourselves.

Set aside some time later in the day for a nap or rest. It can be easier to get going if we know that we can plan on some resting time later. And, if we're not tired, it will seem like a bonus to have the extra time.

If necessary, allow a little extra time in bed to just pull yourself together. Have a book at the bedside or listen to the radio or TV to get started.

If you are still having trouble getting out of bed, consider the possibility of depression. Sometimes sleeping becomes a way of escaping life when it seems too difficult. Depression requires specialized help. Don't be afraid to seek it out. IBD is enough to handle without adding depression to it. Most everyone with IBD suffers from some depression at one time or another. It's no sin to be depressed. But not seeking help is being unfair to yourself and your family.

Notes

Dear Audrey,

I can barely manage my daily chores. It makes me angry that I can't do the "fun" things that others do. I hardly do anything extra anymore. If it's not the diarrhea, I just don't have the energy. I find that I'm afraid to plan ahead for fear that I will not feel well when it's time to go to the party, theater, etc. Is there anything I can do, or do I just have to learn to accept the fact that sports, socializing, travel, or just fun in general are no longer possible? —G.P.

Dear G.P.,

Your feelings have certainly been shared by many of us living with IBD. Although at the beginning it might seem like the pleasures in life aren't possible, we can learn to make adjustments so that we can partake in most activities. Individuals with Crohn's disease and colitis have traveled, participated in sports, attended theaters and concerts, acted in theater groups, taken classes, danced, run, socialized, and enjoyed a fulfilling sexual life. In other columns I have dealt with sexual issues and travel. In this column I would like to share some tips with you to bring additional fun into your life.

The first step is to plan ahead. If you know you have an important evening event, arrange to rest during the day. Allow yourself extra time to get ready so that if you have to keep going to the bathroom, you won't get further frustrated at the thought of being late. You can plan on reading, making a call, or just watching a program if you are done early. If you start out under pressure, it makes everything much more difficult.

Next pack your supplies. Once you have them packed, you can use them for future outings. Depending on how you are feeling, some of the items you may need are extra clothes or just underclothes, medications, special food and something to drink. A plastic juice bottle can be half filled with water, iced tea or any other non-carbonated drink and put in the freezer the night before. When you are ready to leave, just fill the rest and you will have a cold drink with you to avoid dehydration.

Another item that is handy when your energy is limited is a collapsible camp stool, which can be used for rest breaks. It's amazing how many times you could be sitting and waiting instead of standing.

The next step in planning ahead is to find out about bathrooms. Call

ASK AUDREY

ahead, look at seating arrangements in concert halls, ask others. Even if you are not able to do it ahead of time, allow time to check on the bathrooms as soon as you arrive, before it becomes an emergency. Often there are special lavatory facilities that you can negotiate to use by just explaining the situation. For instance, at the outdoor Meadowbrook concerts in Michigan, a nurse is stationed at a bathroom right next to the public bathrooms. If you talk to her ahead of time, you can probably avoid the long lines.

The lack of energy problem can, of course, often be handled by just pacing yourself. However, there are times that pacing alone is not enough. Talk to your doctor about getting permission for a handicapped sticker. Or if even driving seems like too much at times, going in a wheelchair is better than not going at all. Remember, for us this is only a temporary situation.

For some people, there are other issues that make going out and socializing difficult. It's important that we explore to make sure that the illness isn't just masking a problem that needs attention.

It's best to make extra efforts to have fun. Once we are doing something we enjoy, we usually feel better. Start gradually. There may be times when you need to stay home. Even then, if possible, find pleasurable things to do. Pick something easy. As you build your confidence, the activities which once seemed impossible will become easier.

Learning good time and energy management skills will enable you to start enjoying life. Don't look at the fun activities as just something extra. Give them some priority. We won't feel better if life is just work.

So, G.P., don't be afraid to make plans. Just learn the various ways you can modify situations to make fun possible. I know it sounds like a lot of work right now, but take one step at a time. I can guarantee the results are worth it.

<u>Notes</u>

Holidays can be a real source of joy but they also can cause concern for those with IBD. Here are answers to some of the questions I have been asked about coping with the holidays.

How can patients work with friends and family to minimize the stress of preparing for the holidays?

Give yourself more time to prepare. Start long before the holiday actually arrives. Realize that things don't have to be perfect. Consider your expectations. Often we lose sight of the fact that the most important aspect of the holidays is celebrating with loved ones. Everything doesn't have to resemble *Better Homes and Gardens*. Learn time management techniques such as prioritizing, delegating, and, most importantly, saying "no" when necessary.

A person who isn't feeling well may worry that his illness could ruin the holidays for family and friends. If you're going to travel to a big get-together with family or friends and are concerned about having a flare-up, what are the best ways to explain your concerns to the people you're visiting?

Communicate ahead of time. They will feel more comfortable if they know your needs. Let them know if you are on a special diet or have special requirements. Explain that you need to have a bathroom conveniently located.

If your strength is limited at the time, make sure that plans allow adequate time for rest. That's not a bad idea at any time. Do as much as you can for yourself in advance. Have your doctor give you the name of a doctor in the city you plan to visit. Make sure you have a letter from him or her, telling about your condition. If you fly, it's also a good idea to carry medications on the plane and not risk their loss. The most important items to pack are a sense of humor and a pleasant disposition, so that your host and hostess won't mind any inconveniences that may ensue. Incidentally, worrying about a flare-up only makes it more likely to happen. Be prepared in case, but go expecting to enjoy yourself.

ASK AUDREY

73

How can a parent explain the fact that they may be tired or ill in a way that will help children to deal with their disappointment or fears about the parent's health?

Whether it's a holiday or not, the child has to know about a parent's illness. What you tell a child depends on age and sophistication. Remember the child that wanted to know where he came from and whose mother went into a long explanation of the birds and the bees? The child waited patiently and then said, "Johnny comes from Chicago. Where do I come from?"

Try to learn what the child's concerns are. Children are often concerned that you will die, or that the illness may be contagious. Other concerns are that there won't be anybody to take care of them if you are in the hospital.

As far as the holidays go, if you are ill at the time, modify celebrations. Enlist the family to help out. Make it a game. Order in or use frozen food instead of spending long hours in the kitchen. Or instruct the children to do some cooking if they are old enough. Again, remember it is not what you eat that is important, it's celebrating together. Think creatively. If you are confined to bed, make your bedroom the center focus of the holiday festivities.

How do you deal with your own disappointment?

People tend to expect more on the holidays. Movies, books, TV and advertising always depict the so-called perfect family gathering. Even without an illness, most people have difficulty in accepting reality. Our memories often fail us, and we only remember the good times. For some, just being with family is a cause for anxiety. In that case we're disappointed before anything happens because we feel our family doesn't measure up to the standards that we see in the media.

Instead of looking at your limitations during the holidays, look at what you can do. For instance, you'll feel much better if you focus on what you can eat rather than what you can't.

Help someone less fortunate than you are. It's not hard to find someone whose situation is worse than yours. It might just be a phone call to someone shut in, but it will make you feel better as well.

Make sure your expectations are realistic. Remember everything is "time-limited." This time, too, will pass. Talk to someone who wants to listen. Express feelings of disappointment.

Many people become depressed around the holidays. These feelings can be compounded if you're feeling ill, especially when you are alone. How can patients cope?

Patients should plan ahead to try and prevent situations that may cause depression. Modify plans to suit your requirements. Above all, do not leave having company around to chance. Make plans to be with someone. If worse comes to worst, at least use the phone to make contact with others. Again, remember others are lonely on holidays when they can't be with their families. If you can't find ways to relieve the depression, don't hesitate to seek professional help. If possible, try to find someone that has some understanding of the special needs of the physically ill patient.

How can patients cope with being hospitalized during the holiday season?

Nobody wants to be in the hospital for a holiday. However, if it's necessary, make the most out of a distressing situation. Decorate your room. Have your family help. Arrange for your family to visit and perhaps share a holiday meal with you. If you're on I.V.'s and can't eat, use your imagination and sense of humor and pretend it's your turkey dinner. It will be something that you'll remember for a long time, long after you will have remembered any particular meal. If you exchange gifts, use the phone or the mail to buy the gifts and have them delivered to you. Buy yourself a gift too. It doesn't have to be anything expensive, but it's okay to pamper yourself a little. If celebrating the holiday is very important to you, arrange to have a celebration when you get home.

Take control; you decide when and how you want to celebrate. Consider how much more you will appreciate celebrating the holiday next time when you are feeling well.

Notes

PART V:
RELATIONSHIPS

Dear Audrey,

I'm beginning to think that nobody understands me. I've had colitis for three years now, and I'm really getting frustrated. If I tell my husband how I feel, he just tells me to call the doctor or take my medicine. My friends are getting tired of hearing about my bouts. Family members are beginning to think that I'm just trying to avoid family functions. It seems that nobody understands me. Do others feel the way I do? If so, how do they handle it? —F.L.

Dear F.L.,

I hear your frustration and want you to know that you certainly are not alone. There are several aspects of IBD that make it especially difficult for others to understand. One is that this illness is not visible. A broken arm is much easier for people to understand than an invisible illness like IBD.

Another aspect that makes it harder for others to understand is that Crohn's disease and colitis are not consistent. In the case of a broken arm, for instance, it might be slightly different for each person. However, once the arm is broken, except for healing, the changes are usually minimal. Not so with IBD. Not only is each case different, but the reactions can change rapidly. It's hard for people to understand how you can be so sick one moment and then be able to go about normal activities in the same day.

Another factor is the chronicity of IBD. If a person is in an accident, everybody rallies around until the emergency is over. In our society, people are good at responding to emergencies. Unfortunately, after awhile they lose interest. So a chronic illness like IBD frustrates others as well as the individual who has it.

Considering all the above, it's not surprising that you recognize a lack of understanding. Fortunately, there are some steps we can take to see that

ASK AUDREY

we get some of the understanding that is so necessary.

- Start with your husband. Men have been raised to be action-oriented. Your husband is probably feeling frustrated because he feels helpless and wants to find solutions. His way of handling your problems is to suggest something you can do. Communicate with him. Let him know that when you are talking about not feeling well, you are not asking him to do anything. Explain that you just want him to listen and understand. While you're at it, also listen to what he is feeling. Communication skills are so important, but usually they are not taught at school. If you need help there are books, tapes, and even classes on the subject of communication.

- Seek out the Crohn's & Colitis Foundation of America, which offers support groups. They enable you to talk with others that have gone through similar experiences. Here in Michigan we have our annual Coping Conference, usually in May. Although it is just one day, participants have found it extremely helpful to share feelings and learn new ways of coping with IBD.

- Teach those that don't understand about the illness. Those individuals who are important to you need some education. You can tell them about IBD yourself, or you can give them the wonderful educational materials available at the CCFA office. Those that are closest to you could be invited to attend a CCFA meeting or a Coping Conference. This will enable them to have a better understanding of the illness and also open the doors to communication.

- Look for understanding from the general public, although it is still difficult. "How are you?" does not require a dissertation on how many times you went to the bathroom, your stomach cramps, etc. Unfortunately, if you just reported every symptom that occurred, you would soon get the reputation of being a hypochondriac. That doesn't mean that you shouldn't find someone to talk to. It can be a family member or friend, someone from CCFA, a clergyman, doctor or other professional person, or anybody who truly wants to understand.

• Work on becoming a more understanding person yourself. Develop your listening skills. Understanding people attract other understanding people. Individuals who feel understood by you are more willing to reciprocate.

So, F.L., my conclusion is don't give up. Like so many other problems we have to deal with, finding understanding is difficult. It does require effort. However, the results will be worth it.

Notes

Dear Audrey,
I have a child with IBD, and I'm so frustrated. I don't know where to turn. Is there anything that I can do? I feel so helpless. —C.M.

Dear C.M.,

I've received a growing number of requests for counseling from parents of children with *Crohn's* or colitis. Many initially seek help for their child, but then realize that IBD is a disease that affects the entire family. Often the family members' needs are neglected. In this column, I would like to look at the various approaches a parent can use to cope. They are as follows:

PERCEPTUAL: How you view IBD has a lot to do with how well you adjust. If you view it as a disaster, something shameful, or an overwhelming burden that can't be overcome, it will only make matters worse. If you look at it as a challenge, an opportunity to develop new strengths and a source of greater meaning to life, then you're on your way toward more effective coping.

EDUCATIONAL: An important aspect of coping is to gather all the resources available and learn all that you can about the disease. The CCFA has useful printed material as well as excellent educational programs that can help you in this area.

EMOTIONAL: Be aware that you, too, have feelings about the illness: sadness, anger, fear, resentment; many of the same feelings that your child may experience. Get in touch with these feelings. Try to understand them, but most of all, don't displace feelings that belong to you onto your child. You aren't responsible for your child's illness, and you shouldn't expect your child to be responsible for your frustration and other feelings.

SOCIAL: Too often the extra demands on your time start to limit your social life. At this time, it is even more important to have social support from friends. Do let them know how they can help. They, too, are probably feeling helpless and would like to show their concern in some concrete way.

ASK AUDREY

It may be just running an errand or bringing over a dinner, but it will let them be involved.

RECREATIONAL: Parents of children with IBD can easily neglect their own needs because of the extra burdens that are placed on them. It is very important to take time out and have fun. Reward yourself! Do something just for you, whether it's reading a book, taking a swim or just relaxing in a bubble bath. (Note that exercise is a helpful way of handling stress for anyone).

FINANCIAL: Turn to the resources in the community if the financial burden is more than you can handle. A social worker can help you find sources of help. Most community agencies have social workers available, many working on a sliding scale. Make sure you look into insurance for your child for now and the future, and don't overlook scholarship possibilities for schooling.

PHILOSOPHICAL: People who have a purpose in life cope best. Some people find this in religion, others in a cause. Working for a cure for IBD with CCFA has been an excellent way many parents have learned to cope (as well as getting the side benefits of support from others facing similar difficulties). Which goal or purpose you choose is an individual matter. Having one is the important factor.

FAMILIAL: Roles in the family may change as needs change. New responsibilities may emerge. Siblings without the disease also need attention. Any problems that the family experienced before the illness are further accentuated by the stress of the illness. Flexibility, communication, cooperation and caring are all important goals.

Having a child or any other family member with IBD can be very difficult. It isn't something that can be covered in one article. The best we can do is to accept the situation, not give up hope, develop a sense of humor, and then grow from the experience of a new challenge. This attitude can serve as an example to our children, so that instead of looking at IBD as a disaster and giving up, they too can turn it into a growth experience and develop skills that will be useful all their lives.

Notes

Dear Audrey,

My husband is having a great deal of difficulty with his colitis. I think that he could use some help from a psychologist, but he gets angry when I even bring up the subject. I don't understand. He goes to the doctor when his body hurts, and he goes to the dentist when his teeth hurt. Now he's hurting emotionally, but just the suggestion that he seek help infuriates him. —E.W.

Dear E.W.,

I hear this story frequently from spouses, parents and even children who are concerned about their loved ones and frustrated by their unwillingness to seek help. Let's try to understand their reluctance. In the 1950's colitis was labeled a psychosomatic illness; it was postulated that specific personality patterns related to the illness. Today, no one who studies colitis believes it is caused by "nerves" or specific personality traits. However, many haven't kept up with the latest research and continue to worry that the disease is caused solely by psychological factors. Often their reaction to this concern is to completely deny their feelings. The effect of this denial is the ignoring of the proven role of stress in all illnesses.

All illnesses can cause stress, and most illnesses can be exacerbated by stress. It's understandable why patients may need to deny that emotions might be involved. The idea of psychotherapy can be scary. There is a fear of the unknown, and as bad as things may be, there is also a fear of change.

Those with colitis or Crohn's disease have additional concerns. Just having an illness is a narcissistic blow. They feel vulnerable and somewhat diminished compared to how they felt previously. If they believe that seeing a psychologist means admitting they are emotionally disturbed, it's no wonder they find it difficult to do. They are trying to do everything they can to preserve their integrity and self-esteem. Unfortunately, they often view seeing a psychologist as a blow to their self-esteem, as a sign of weakness rather than a sign of strength and a desire to better cope with their illness.

I hope I have given you some idea of the reasons for your husband not seeking help, even when it's probably needed. However, you may understand what worries him but still feel frustrated. You might consider seeking therapy for yourself to deal with your own feelings. This will serve two purposes.

ASK AUDREY

The direct benefit is that you will be working on your present feelings. A side benefit will be that, by obtaining therapy for yourself, you will take some of the stigma and fear out of therapy for your spouse. Eventually, this may make it easier for him to seek help.

Notes

Dear Audrey,

Before I got sick, my husband and I got along fine. Now we are constantly fighting and he seems so angry. It's hard enough for me to deal with the illness, and he makes it even worse. —C.S.

Dear C.S.,

Often couples faced with IBD will experience some marital disharmony if they are not aware of some of the problems that can occur.

Peter Martin[1] lists several values inherent in a healthy marriage. These include:

- The capacity of each individual to stand alone, to be independent.

- The capacity of being supportive of the mate and accepting support from the mate in time of need.

- The capacity for emotional intimacy, physical intimacy and adequate sexual intercourse.

Let's look at how illness interacts with them:

When we are sick there are times that it is difficult to be independent. Physically we may be too weak to do things on our own. However, we must remember that even at these times there is nothing wrong with our minds, and it is possible to be more independent by using them. One of the most independent people I ever knew was completely flat on his back and couldn't move at all. Yet he maintained complete control of his life.

When we are feeling terrible we want others to support us, but we sometimes forget that they, too, have problems and need support. They may be worried about what is going to happen and feel helpless. They may be upset about the changes in their life. Anger may be used to cover up these feelings of fear and helplessness. It becomes extremely important to give your spouse emotional support and try to listen to his or her feelings.

Often, when we need it, we find it hard to accept support. Physical illness is a wound to our self-esteem. To make up for it, we think we have to be better than human and do everything ourselves. Many women I have seen are doing more housework than normal. Sometimes we don't accept our spouse's support because we don't like the way they do things. We need to learn that if we're asking someone else to do something for us, it's best to let them do it their way and not fret about it.

The capacity for emotional intimacy can be hindered by holding back on communication. The wife doesn't want to get the husband angry and the husband doesn't want to get the wife upset. Pretty soon they aren't talking about any conflictual matters. Since many of our important feelings may evoke conflict, we shut down and don't talk to each other, and emotional intimacy goes out the window.

When we are feeling sick, unattractive or bothered with diarrhea, we may not feel like having sexual intercourse. But, we can still give pleasure to our partners. We may even get in the mood ourselves. Regardless, it's important not to stop physical intimacy. Physical intimacy is a lot more than just intercourse. It is touching, holding, cuddling, stroking and all of those good things that make a couple feel closer to each other.

Obviously I can't cover the entire subject of marital conflict in one column. The important aspects, though, are to try to understand where your partner is coming from, learn to communicate, and then look to see what you can accomplish.

We can't make other people change, but we can change, and when we do, they often change in response to our changes. Something else to remember is that the stress of illness will bring out a lot of problems that might have always been there but are now accentuated. In that event, you should consider obtaining help so these issues won't be a continuous interference with your life!

[1] Martin, MD, Peter A., "A Marital Therapy Manual", (Brunner/Mazel, Publishers, New York, NY, 1976)

<u>Notes</u>

Dear Audrey,

My wife and I are always fighting, and it seems every time we have a fight, I get upset and then get sick. I don't know if you can help me, but suggestions would be appreciated. —N.R.

Dear N.R.,

Congratulations. You have already taken two steps towards solving the problem. First, you have identified the connection between becoming upset and getting sick. We don't know what causes IBD, but more and more evidence is showing that emotional upsets play a part in exacerbating most illnesses.

Second, you have decided to ask for help, and that's often very difficult to do. An illness can put extra stress on a marriage. For example, there are additional demands upon time and money. The uncertainty of the "time bomb" effect can wreak havoc with a couple's social life. In addition, many spouses stop communicating because they are afraid to upset their partner and make matters worse. These stresses can affect a couple's sexual life (see letters on sexuality).

The above concerns are IBD-associated. However, every married couple has normal problems dealing with in-laws, household duties, raising children, finances, etc.

Let me give you a few hints that might help ease some of the tensions around your house.

- If something your wife does upsets you, tell her what you are feeling instead of accusing her. "I was worried when you were late" will open up conversation. "You never get anywhere on time" will just lead to an argument.

- Try to understand what your wife is feeling. What's bothering her? Have you touched upon an issue that's sensitive to her?

- See if you can figure out what the fight is really about. Are you both just tired? Is there some issue that you haven't talked about that is the real culprit causing dissension?

ASK AUDREY

- Don't try to avoid fights at all cost. Instead, learn how to fight fairly. Don't call each other names. Stick to the issue and work on a resolution. If it's not an important issue to you, you can let it go; or you can compromise; or, finally, you can just agree to disagree.

- If either one of you is so upset you can't control your emotions, give yourself a cooling off time. However, do make sure that you designate a time to resolve the issue.

- Read some books on relationships. The library is full of them. One book to start with is *You Just Don't Understand* by Deborah Tannen. (References to this book and others are listed in the column on reading material)

- Don't be afraid to talk to a member of the clergy or to a marriage counselor. Somebody less emotionally involved can add a fresh view to the situation.

Remember, all couples have fights. The fight itself is not the problem, unless, of course, there is physical abuse. The problem arises when you avoid the issues rather than work them out.

Notes

Dear Audrey,

I'm 23 years old and have ileitis. I'm feeling very discouraged. I'm afraid nobody will want to marry me with this disease. I'm having a difficult time finding dates, let alone a marriage partner. Do people with IBD date, get married and have normal family lives? —J.F.

Dear J.F.,

Of course people with colitis and ileitis can have normal family lives. However, it is common to hear of single people with IBD, young and old alike, who feel that nobody will want them. I like to look at this issue from two perspectives: that of the individual and that of the possible mate.

As far as the individual goes, hard questions must be asked: "Would I be a desirable mate without my IBD? Do I like myself? What are my strong points? Do I have a good sense of humor? Am I a caring person? Do I listen and speak well? Am I intelligent? Do I have good common sense?"

The list is endless. If we really think about it, we probably already have many strong points that can be enhanced. Sometimes I hear the complaint that someone is too skinny or too fat, too short or too tall, etc. It's important to do the best we can with what we have. It's always amazing to learn what others find attractive. Sometimes physical features that we consider a liability can actually be an asset. Even the illness itself affects others in diverse ways. One person may find it overwhelming; another, a challenge. What is of prime importance is how we feel about ourselves.

We need not let our weaknesses get us down. We all have weaknesses, but trying to do something about them is an attractive quality to many people. For instance, is the illness the only thing we have to talk about? It's important to be an interesting person. Sometimes I hear, "That's fine for people that feel better, but I'm sick and in bed a lot." That's still no excuse for becoming dull. Our body may be sick, but IBD doesn't stop us from thinking.

These days, through radio and television, news and special events are brought directly to us. Certainly we can expand our horizons by reading. If reading is difficult, libraries now offer books on tape. The phone can be used as another connection to the outside world. (See the column about "Thinking Independently.")

ASK AUDREY

However, most of us *can* get out, and it's important to pursue activities in which we are interested. It can be theater, arts, sports, politics, photography, cooking, church or synagogue activities, travel, organizations, literature or even card games. Whatever our interests, there are usually classes or clubs where people with similar interests enjoy themselves while increasing their opportunities for meeting people.

Obviously, there are many ways to improve ourselves that go beyond the scope of this particular column. However, there are many books and tapes available that can help us over some problem areas. Sometimes it takes professional help to help us look at things in a different way. Whatever the way, we have to remember that we take medicine to make our bodies stronger, and we have to pay some attention to the social and personal sides of ourselves as well.

Now, suppose we are doing everything we can to make ourselves desirable partners, and are taking part in activities to meet people, but we still run into disappointment. Perhaps we find someone that won't accept our illness. Unfortunately, there are some people that want perfection in their partners. We should feel lucky to find that out ahead of time. These same people are the ones that would leave when any sickness came up; and sooner or later, everyone has to deal with illness of some kind. These are the people that would not be able to deal with any of the normal kinds of problems that come up during a marriage. They probably would have a hard time dealing with a mate who became less attractive or even coping with the inevitable aging process. How lucky we are to have a screening device to save us the misery of getting involved with them to begin with.

On the other hand, the partner that accepts us with our illness is someone who loves us in spite of it. We know that it's someone who cares about us as a person, and we have a much better chance of making the marriage work.

So, J.F., stop worrying about finding someone. Find yourself. Make yourself strong. Someone who can fully appreciate your strengths will find you.

<u>Notes</u>

Dear Audrey,

I'm writing because it upsets me to see letters like the one J.F. wrote in your Nov.-Dec. '87 column. The letter was written by a young female with ileitis who said "nobody will ever love me because of my disease."

I'm 32 years old and found out about my ileitis eight years ago. Two years ago, I had to have a colostomy. Within a week after surgery I was filing for divorce. Not because of my disease or the surgery, but because my husband kept telling me I was worthless and no one else would ever "put up" with my illness.

He had me believing it for years.

I spent my marriage trying to "make up" for having ileitis, as if it were my choice. Within a few days of my surgery, he was complaining about the inconvenience of running to and from the hospital and how I had to hurry and get back to work because we needed the money for bills. He was on a voluntary lay-off for the past five months and my sick pay and his unemployment checks were covering the bills.

I suggested that he didn't have to visit as often and he accused me of having an affair only four days after surgery. I called a lawyer. My husband told me again that no one would ever want me. I said, "I know, but being alone or lonely has got to be better than living in this hell."

With no children, I made it as quick as possible. I got my own apartment and for six months hibernated, crying only to my sister and best friend when I became too lonely. I was afraid of meeting a man. He might ask for a date, then another, and it could lead to intimacy, then he'd find out about me and run. That would hurt even more.

Then, I made a new friend at work and began going out with her and some other single women. I hated it at first, but I kept going because it was killing me to hide in my little apartment and I knew it. We went to the same place every couple of weeks. I'd sit in the corner all nervous and watch as my new friends got asked to dance and talked to their friends there.

Slowly, I started to make friends and relax. I started going there just to talk to the friends I had made, not to meet men, and pretty soon I had no problem finding dates. I became a loving and caring person, which also helped me spot the users and the losers quicker.

ASK AUDREY

I've met some terrific people, some great guys; a few have been lovers, but none have ever considered my ostomy or disease a problem or handicap, because I don't. The best I can do is help them understand it and show them I can live with it.

I've been the one to break off any relationships, usually because of insecurities they had about themselves. I'm still friends with them. They've all told me that I'm the only person they could really open up to. I care about people and their feelings and always will because there are too many people who don't. I could easily just take anyone who'd take me, but I found out the hard way that feeling proud to be me is a lot more important than being married just because some guy is willing to. Tell J.F. to go out and make friends first, and if it's God's will, the right guy will come along. If she sets up her own life with a job, goals, plans, and friends to make her happy, chances are some nice guy will come along to mess up the plans by making her all "starry-eyed" and confused. Life's funny that way. —D.D.

Dear D.D.,

What a joy and inspiration it was to receive your letter. It certainly shows that we don't have to let ileitis or even an ostomy keep us from making the most of our lives. With your permission, I am publishing your letter in full so that others can be encouraged by your experience and courage. Thank you so much for sharing it.

Notes

Dear Audrey,

I'm planning on getting married soon, and I'm concerned that my Crohn's disease might affect my sexual life. Is it possible to have a normal sex life? What kinds of sexual problems do individuals with IBD experience?

—B.L.

Dear B.L.,

Congratulations on your upcoming marriage. I'm glad that you asked about the sexual implications of IBD. People find this is a difficult area to talk about and there is often needless misunderstanding because of the lack of communication.

The simple answer to your question is that, usually, IBD does *not* prevent us from having a very satisfactory sex life. But, there are possible problem areas that could cause you or others some concern in the future:

- **The general symptoms of the illness.** Pain, fatigue, nausea and diarrhea—the most common culprits with IBD patients—can impede your sex life when you are experiencing these symptoms. However, with good communication and some planning, these problems *can* be overcome. Fatigue can certainly put a damper on sexual activity. But, with a little planning, it's possible to find the times that you feel the strongest. It's hard to think about sex when you are in pain, nauseous or experiencing diarrhea (although some find that sex can divert attention away from the pain), but the way you handle these symptoms is very important. Here's where communication plays an important role. Love, caring and sexuality can be expressed in many ways besides intercourse. You know how. Sometimes, you just forget.

- **The psychological impact of the illness.** This can include depression, altered sense of identity, body image changes, loss of job, and role changes within the family and society. Certainly sexual relations are strained when you feel depressed or concerned about your body image, your role in the family, or your work. What happens in these areas will have impact in the bedroom. It's important to involve family members with your concerns because they, too, will have feelings about what's going on. Spouses may be concerned that they are going to cause you to be sicker, or that they may harm you in some way. Others feel selfish that they have needs as well. Communication, again, is the key word. How you look, how you speak, how you act, and most of all how you feel and care can contribute to your sexual attractiveness.

Some fear that they will be unattractive or rejected if they have to have an ostomy or if they gain weight as a result of prednisone. These fears may accompany a fear of abandonment. Ostomy surgery need not interfere with sexual activity. The United Ostomy Organization offers excellent literature on sex and ostomies. Again, I can't repeat enough that a person who loves you won't be bothered by physical changes. Why would you bother with a person who doesn't love you?

• **Specific fears about sex and IBD**. There are all kinds of concerns about sex, with or without IBD. These concerns have to be dealt with as they normally would. You have to work on them, or, if you run into an impasse, you should seek professional help.

Additionally, there are specific fears for those with IBD. Included are fears that sexual activity will provoke symptoms, or that one's sex life cannot be resumed. Some fear that sex will make the illness worse. Some fear pregnancy. (The CCFA has an excellent pamphlet on pregnancy). In all cases, it is important to get the proper information and talk with your doctor about your concerns. Also consult your doctor so you know if any of the medications you are taking could affect your sex drive.

Another less serious but more embarrassing problem is that of the possibility of having an accident during intercourse. True, it can be embarrassing, but one has to remember that your partner loves you and is more concerned about *your* reaction. How you handle the situation makes a great deal of difference. You can get hysterical and hate your body and lower your self image, or you can look at it as unfortunate, but something that happened. Your doctor may be able to prescribe medication that can make you feel more secure during intimate times.

In all situations, it's important to focus on the potential, not the limitations. Realize that sex is expressed in many ways. Think of the whole person rather than just the genitals. Flexibility, communication, education, understanding, and humor are all important. Above all, you should try to do what you can to improve any difficulties in your sexual relationship, and never abandon the idea that you *can* do something to enrich this important aspect of your life.

Notes

Other questions asked regarding sexuality:

What are the most common concerns about sexuality among newly diagnosed adult IBD patients?

A newly-diagnosed patient is faced with the uncertainty of what life will be like physically, socially and psychologically. What physical changes are going to take place? Will there be limitations? How will it affect social life? Psychologically there can be many reactions. Some people will become depressed. Some will suffer from low self-esteem or become concerned about their body image.

How do the concerns of single patients differ from those of married people?

A married person wonders if a spouse will still find him or her attractive. Will they be able to have children? How will their sex life be affected by the illness? Single people have the same concerns but are also worried that nobody will want to be involved with them because of their illness.

Are there important differences in the way men and women view the disease's impact on sexuality?

Basically both are concerned about their partner's reactions. A man may feel less masculine if he's out of work or needs care. However, today the roles of men and women are less rigid and role reversal is not the problem it once was. There is still some residue of a man's needing to feel "macho" and able to perform, and a woman wondering if she will be attractive enough to be desirable. I prefer to think that these are individual reactions. I do notice a difference in the spouses. Women seem to adapt to the caretaking role more readily than men do. Women are taught to nurture from an earlier age.

What suggestions would you make to help single IBD patients feel more comfortable about dating and sexual relationships? For instance, how

and when do you decide to tell someone you're dating about the disease?

I wrote a whole column on singles' concerns (see "Finding a Spouse"). As far as when to tell someone about your illness is concerned, it's important to let the person know as soon as you sense that the relationship is more than casual. It's not necessarily the first thing you would say. Telling someone you have some health problems may be a start. It is important to explain what IBD is and how it affects you. Going to a meeting or sharing CCFA literature with your date can be helpful. The important issue is how you present IBD. If you seem overwhelmed, others will be too. If you can take the disease in stride, you may find that others can as well.

What advice would you give a couple who are hoping to have children?

Most couples have no difficulty conceiving, however infertility may be a problem. Sulfasalazine can cause infertility in men, and severe IBD sometimes results in infertility in both men and women.

In that situation all avenues should be considered. Infertility specialists now have many new methods available. If conception isn't possible, adoption is also an alternative. Children bond with the parents who raise them. Adoption procedures should be started as soon as possible, since it sometimes requires a very long time. If the above steps are impossible, there are still other options to bring love to a child's life. You might try foster children, participate in big brother or sister programs, or find an individual child or group of children that would benefit from your caring about them.

Some people who have IBD may avoid sexual relationships because of self-consciousness about their illness. What advice can you give to such patients?

Sexual relationships are an important aspect of being a whole person. Before you rule out this side of your life, it might be advisable to seek professional help. On the lighter side, it helps to remember that most people are self-conscious about sexual relationships. People are always wondering what others think about them. If they aren't dealing with an illness, they may be dealing with some difficulties in how they perceive their body. They may feel that they are too fat, too thin, too short, too tall, etc.

If a patient is having difficulty coping sexually, at what point should he consider getting professional help? What does the therapy entail?

If you are feeling anger, guilt, resentment, depression or lack of self-esteem and are having difficulty dealing with these feelings yourself, therapy could be useful. A simple guideline is to notice if you are feeling unhappy and if you feel helpless to do anything about it. Then it may be time to talk to a professional. The first step is seeing somebody for an evaluation. Sometimes treatment may be limited to sex therapy, where you learn techniques to help you work out sexual problems. Sometimes there are other issues in the marriage. If there were even slight problems before, illness can exacerbate them. In this case, a marriage counselor might be indicated. Most often when there are problems, it is a result of individual issues that require someone trained in understanding individual dynamics; why we act the way we do. The same therapist might be skilled in all three, but the emphasis is different. Organizations[1] can be called upon to recommend credentialed therapists in your area. Hospitals and universities can also be helpful. You can ask friends; or sometimes your local chapter has therapists who are aware of the special needs of patients with IBD. In all of the above therapies, it is important that the therapist understand IBD and what part that plays in the difficulties. The main purpose of therapy is to help you understand what's preventing you from accomplishing what you desire.

What is the role of a support group in helping patients deal with sexuality and IBD?

Support groups enable a person to know that he or she is not alone. Also it adds to everyone's self-esteem to be able to help someone else. Support groups aid in obtaining information and in giving encouragement. Just talking about issues can sometimes alleviate stress.

[1] **The following organizations have specific requirements for membership. For more information write or call:**

American Association for Marriage and Family Therapy
1133 15th Street NW
Washington, DC 20005
(202) 452-0109

American Association of Sex Educators, Counselors, and Therapists
P.O. Box 238
Mount Vernon, VA 52314
(319) 895-8407

American Group Psychotherapy Association
25 East 21st Street-6th Floor
New York, NY 10010
(212) 477-2677

Notes

Dear Audrey,
One of the concerns that I have is how to make and keep friends when I have an illness like IBD. Sometimes I find it easier to just not see people. —R.K.

Dear R.K.,
Friends are very important, especially so if you have a chronic illness. There are many ways to make and maintain friendships despite the limitations of IBD. Let's look at some of them.

- Friends want to help you but, not knowing how, they may say nothing and not call or come around. Your communication skills will have to be better. Learning how to share feelings often opens the way for better communication.

- Let your friends help you. They may feel helpless too. They may want to do something, but not know what. Asking them to do a small task can relieve their sense of helplessness. You may need a ride to the doctor, a dinner brought in, or just a phone call or visit. It makes them feel better to do something specific and concrete.

- It's tempting when something is hurting you to tell everybody all the details. You can get a reputation as a hypochondriac. Others are interested for awhile, but they become uncomfortable when you elaborate too often. If every time they ask how you feel you say, "My stomach hurts, etc.," eventually they'll stop asking. It is important to be able to share these feelings with some people, but be selective. Make sure they really want to hear.

- Be an interesting person. You cannot blame people for not wanting to be around if your digestive system is the only topic of conversation. Read the newspaper. Listen to talk shows. Become aware of the world around you. Remember that you are not just an illness; you are a person with all kinds of ideals, values, etc.

ASK AUDREY

• Be a friend. If we want friends, we have to care about others and be considerate of their needs. During times when we are feeling better, it's important to help friends out. Be supportive.

• Accept your friends and their flaws. Nobody's perfect. We are looking for acceptance, and we have to learn to be more accepting. Talk about problem areas. Try to identify how the problems make you feel and what can be done.

• Get involved in organizations. Help others that are less fortunate. You will not only have more interesting causes to talk about, but you might even meet some people along the way. CCFA is a great place to start.

• Make an effort to keep your social appointments and to be prompt. This can be very difficult with IBD. Allow yourself extra time and plan to rest if necessary.

• Instead of saying, "I can't go," make the situation one you can handle. Again, use your creativity. Sometimes advance planning like checking out the bathroom, making special arrangements for food, being dropped off at the door, etc., can make you comfortable.

• Take the initiative with social activities. Don't stand on ceremony waiting for someone to call you. There is someone that would be happy to hear from you right now!

Your medical treatment is very important, but don't underestimate the power of your friends. Good friends are treasures that will help you through some of the more difficult times. Work on finding and keeping a circle of friends.

<u>Notes</u>

FAMILY REACTIONS
by Lawrence Kron, Ph.D.

A s patients and other family members read the articles that have preceded this, they will note that the focus is primarily upon the illness and the trials of the patient who has to deal with it. It is appropriate that our attention be directed toward the patient, in the first instance. However, there is a potential for unnecessary stresses and strains to occur if the needs of other family members are ignored, and this is often the case. The purpose of this article is to briefly outline some of the problems faced by family members as they attempt to cope with a chronic illness in their family.

One of the first difficulties family members confront is the anxiety engendered by not knowing what is going on with the patient. This problem parallels the patient's own concerns, e.g., "What's wrong with me (her, him)?" "What can be done?" "Will it be debilitating, or fatal?", etc. Family members both want answers and don't want them at the same time. Responses vary from totally ignoring the condition and expecting the patient to function exactly as before to a hand-wringing over-concern and over-solicitousness of every need of the patient. At either extreme such a response is highly detrimental to the family relationships. Ignoring the problem contributes to the patient's sense of having failed the family and often produces a desire in the patient to compensate by trying to do more than is physically or emotionally healthy, with potentially dire consequences. On the other hand, to be over-involved with the patient contributes to infantilization of the patient, adds to an already lowered self-esteem and produces a slowly growing resentment in the family members.

The more healthy approach by family members includes education, communication and involvement. Most anxiety and reactions to it are the consequence of "not knowing". Family members should be as conversant with the patient's diagnosis, treatment, and prognosis as is the patient. A sharing of information between patient and family members is a necessity. This includes family members sharing their own feelings and concerns about whatever is on their minds, not just the illness. The patient may have a chronic illness but is not helpless or incompetent. Being of help to family members usually has a salutary effect upon patients.

ASK AUDREY

Finally, family members need to be involved in the illness itself, but only in ways that are useful from the patient's point of view. To do things for the patient, which he or she could do on his or her own, will at best be frustrating to the patient, who has a need to be productive. To refuse help when the patient is helpless will send a message that the family can't tolerate the illness. The family members need to distinguish these situations. Helping when help is truly needed, and backing off when it is not, are both kindnesses to the patient.

Looking back at these few paragraphs one can notice how easy it is to gravitate to a focus on the patient's concerns. Family members need to be constantly aware of their own needs and concerns. The patient may not be able to contribute as in the past, resulting in family members' energies being over-taxed. So the family members need to be sure to program into their routine such time as they need to "recharge their batteries." Failure to do so will result in a growing resentment, which will seep out in one's mannerisms, tone of voice, etc., all to the detriment of family harmony.

It's important to remember that, as family members, you count too. Your emotional comfort and well-being needs just as much nurturing as does the patient's. In the long run, tending adequately to your own needs will make you a happier, more pleasant person to be with, and this is the best atmosphere for the growth of healthy family relationships.

Notes

PART VI:
EMOTIONS AND IBD

Dear Audrey,

Since I have had Crohn's disease, I have experienced so many different feelings that I'm beginning to wonder if I'm abnormal. Please let me know if others also experience mood swings.   —P.G.

Dear P.G.,

Every human being experiences a wide range of feelings, all depending upon the circumstances.   In fact, each day is filled with a variety of them. After the onset of an illness such as inflammatory bowel disease, it is quite common for one's emotions to be stirred up.   Medicines, like prednisone, may also cause mood swings.   Each individual is different, but there are some strong feelings which we all share:

- **Fear**. There may be fears about how the illness will affect work, school, or the future in general. Some of us worry that we will lose the love of our family and friends. Others are afraid of pain, or the side effects from medication, hospitalization, and testing procedures.

- **Anger**. "Why me?" is a common question. Sometimes the anger is directed against fate, but often it gets displaced to people that we are close to, and our family life is disrupted.

- **Guilt**. Even though we do not know the cause of these diseases, we often feel that we have done something to contribute to the onset of the illness. Even if that's not a concern, there may be guilty feelings for the extra burden that illness imposes on the family.

- **Shame**. In our society we downplay and ignore anything that has to do with bathroom habits. The whole world goes to the bathroom, but

ASK AUDREY

people with IBD often feel shame because they have a disease that has to do with the bowels.

- **Depression**. At times we feel like everything is going wrong. Life seems overwhelming, and it becomes difficult to believe that things will get better. We get down on ourselves and add to the burdens of the illness.

- **Frustration**. Sometimes our bodies do not react in the way that we would like. We find we can't do everything we'd like. We become frustrated.

- **Alienation**. There are times when we feel very alone. It seems as if no one can understand what we are feeling.

None of these feelings are abnormal. Recognize that there are all kinds of feelings we may experience. If we recognize our feelings, we will be able to talk to others about them. This is an important part of the process of learning to accept them.

Notes

Dear Audrey,

In the last issue of the CCFA Newsletter (Sept/Oct, 1988), a review stated that IBD is *not* related to stress. I disagree with this. Could you please tell me if my thinking and my family physician are wrong. The review rebutted an article that originally appeared in the April, 1988, issue of *Good Housekeeping* magazine. Thank you. —N.K.

Dear N.K.

I'm glad that you questioned the remarks about the *Good Housekeeping* article. The review criticized the article for perpetuating the "myth" that IBD is caused by stress. A careful reading discloses the review to be in error, not the article. The article states: "Today, we know that psychological factors play a role in all illnesses, although in some more than others. We have also learned that there is no such thing as a pure psychosomatic disease, one caused solely by stress. Stress alone cannot damage body tissue. It is how we cope with stress in our mind and how our body reacts in the process that determines whether or not we get sick. If we do become ill, our genes, environment, lifestyle, and other factors determine with what type of disease."

The article also points out that prolonged stress can actually weaken a body's immune system and may make it vulnerable to a host of illnesses. It ends by saying that some physicians welcome the challenge and will work carefully with a patient to identify and treat both the physical and emotional components of an illness. The chart that accompanies the article lists several illnesses, including IBD. It specifies what can be done about the stress and what can be done medically, not stating a preferred treatment. But, in keeping with the theme of the article, it suggests that attention to both mind and body would be helpful. The article is written by Dr. Marvin Stein, professor of psychiatry and chairman of the Department of Psychiatry at the Mount Sinai School of Medicine in New York, who is also past president of the American Psychosomatic Society. He knows what he is writing about. More important than this particular article is the whole stigma attached to the word "psychosomatic." I certainly can appreciate how stressful it is to have people equate "psychosomatic" with being emotionally unstable. However, that is not the case. The meaning of psychosomatic refers to the integration of the mind and the body. In light of all the current research, we would be like

ASK AUDREY

119

ostriches to think that our mind and body are not connected. We see evidence every day. For example, when we give a speech, our body reacts to our stress, and our palms become clammy, or we feel butterflies in our stomachs. People without IBD will develop diarrhea and/or nausea when faced with a difficult situation. So, why should we become immune to body reactions when we have IBD? After all, our bowels are already sensitive.

We could write letters of protest to *Good Housekeeping*, asking them to make the line read: "*Sometimes* it is how we cope with stress in our mind and how our body reacts in the process that *may* determine whether or not we get sick." But we should also be writing letters to CCFA to encourage them to do research in the mind/body connection. Denying the relationship between stress and IBD may make us more comfortable in the short run, but it does great disservice in the long run. Once and for all, let's accept the fact that stress makes a difference in regard to *all* illnesses, and that IBD is no exception. This can be an exciting and encouraging avenue to explore. We can start by reading the article. Think about it: if stress contributes to the effect of IBD, then by understanding what is stressful to us, and learning to better cope with it, we can have a significant impact in reducing the effect. More effectively dealing with stress won't cure IBD all by itself, but it may alleviate a great deal of unnecessary suffering.

Notes

When Psychotherapy is Appropriate

Despite growing public awareness and the educational efforts of CCFA, the outdated attitude still persists that digestive disease is caused by "emotions" or "stress." The scientists and doctors currently studying the disease do not believe that the primary cause of IBD is emotionally based.

The CCFA publication "Questions & Answers About Emotional Factors in Crohn's and Colitis" addresses the question: "Do emotional factors play any part at all in the course of inflammatory bowel disease?" Answer: Body and mind are inseparable and are interrelated in numerous and complex ways. It has been observed that flare-ups of inflammatory bowel disease may occur at the time of an attack of viral or other infectious illness. It also appears likely that some flare-ups of the disease can be triggered by nervous tension or by emotionally stressful life situations. However, this flare-up effect should be carefully separated from the primary cause of inflammatory bowl disease, which is not emotionally based. This publication can be obtained by calling the Michigan Chapter office (810-737-0900) or the national office (800-932-2423).

It is recognized that living with a chronic illness can add stress to our lives. CCFA chapters in some areas of the country have developed support groups that are not professionally led but are mutual help groups that provide a support network for patients with IBD and their families.

However, some situations may require more than a support group. Then therapy should be considered.

Some questions you may want to ponder are:

Why would a person with IBD want therapy?

The burdens of our daily living can at times seem overwhelming to anyone. Adding the burden of a chronic illness adds to the stress. One purpose of therapy is to help us respond to stressful situations more effectively and thereby ease the burden.

What are the concerns of people with IBD?

Some of the more common concerns relate to diet, medication, hospitalization, surgery, tests, and the uncertainty of the illness. Added to this are many interpersonal concerns, such as how the illness affects relationships with family and friends or conditions at work and school. Concerns about the bathroom are almost universally shared.

Is stress the same for everybody?

No. What is stressful for one person may not be for another. Sometimes we are not even aware that something is stressful unless we explore it further.

Why therapy for people with IBD? Doesn't everybody have to deal with stress?

Yes, and it would be helpful for everyone to learn more effective ways to deal with life's stresses. However, the consequences for people with IBD can be more severe, and therefore managing stress is more crucial.

Why is group therapy often recommended?

A group offers the unique opportunity to share feelings with others who understand some of the problems an individual with IBD experiences. It helps a person feel less alone. It provides an opportunity to see how others cope. Sometimes others can express feelings that you have experienced but may not have been able to articulate. There is also the satisfaction of being able to help others. In addition, groups allow us to deal with areas of concern in a safe environment, giving us the skills and insight to be able to apply these methods in the "outside" world. This safe environment is also conducive to the expression of feelings that are better let out than held in, where they could possibly exacerbate the illness.

Regardless of whether it's by self examination, reading, talking, support groups, or individual or group therapy, taking care of your emotional well-being is an important part of your total health care.

Notes

PART VII:
COPING
TECHNIQUES

Dear Audrey,

I get frustrated when I run into a problem. I notice that when things seem out of control, I start to run to the bathroom and it just makes matters worse. Is there any way that you can help? —T.T.

Dear T.T.,

You're not the only one that has encountered some sort of physical symptoms when you run into a problem or feel out of control. However, you must realize that you always have some control of the situation even when you think you don't. There are three aspects of the situation that you can do something about.

First, you can try to *change the circumstances*. If you are bothered by something, such as feeling anxious when you go to the theater, you can arrange for aisle seats. If you have to be away from home, you can take extra clothing or medication with you to make yourself more comfortable.

You can also learn how to handle something disagreeable in a more effective way. Being imaginative, you can listen to music or books on tape while you are going through an unpleasant test. You can learn time management techniques to save time and energy. And you can gain more information to help you feel more comfortable.

Next, you can *work on your relationships*. Everything seems better when you have a good support system. This requires work. Here you have to brush up on your relationship skills. You have to know what it means to be a good friend before you can expect to have good friends. And, you have to know how to get along with family members before you get upset at them.

When you have tried the other two methods and still are faced with a problem, your last resource is to *change your attitude*. Remember that you

ASK AUDREY

always have control of how you view things. You can choose to simply consider the source, ignore it, think that it could be worse, realize that this, too, will pass, or use humor.

These are starters, T.T. Begin to look at your problems as a way of increasing your abilities to cope. You will discover that this will give you the control that you desire.

Notes

Dear Readers,

One of the problems many of us share is that we have unrealistic expectations. We have enough to contend with in dealing with the illness, but then we put unnecessary additional stress on our lives. Albert Ellis called some of these expectations "irrational ideas."[1]

I'll share with you a few of these "irrational ideas" which are the source of many coping difficulties. The sooner we realize that they are irrational, the sooner we can get on with coping.

- First, there's the idea that it is a dire necessity for an adult human being to be loved or approved of by virtually every significant other person in his community.

- Next, there's the idea that one should be thoroughly competent, adequate, and achieving in all possible respects, if one is to consider oneself worthwhile. (This is an idea we see often.)

- Third is the idea that it is awful and catastrophic when things are not the way one would very much like them to be.

- Fourth is the idea that it is easier to avoid than to face certain life difficulties and self responsibilities.

- Fifth is the idea that one should be dependent on others and that one needs someone stronger than oneself on whom to rely.

- Finally, there is the idea that there is invariably a right, precise, and perfect solution to human problems, and that it is catastrophic if this perfect solution is not found.

We can surely see how harboring some of these beliefs can be detrimental to our health. Let us hope that we can recognize them, address them and eventually eliminate this needless source of stress. High expectations are admirable, but keep them rational.

ASK AUDREY

129

[1]Ellis, Albert. <u>A New Guide to Rational Living.</u> Prentice-Hall, Englewood Cliffs, N.J., (1975).

<u>Notes</u>

Dear Audrey,

I live in a very small town where there is no CCFA chapter. I have colitis and I sometimes have great difficulty dealing with it. I feel so isolated. Do you have any suggestions?   —W.L.

Dear W.L.,

You have already taken the first step by reading the CCFA bulletin. You will feel less isolated when you learn that others have similar experiences.

Next, find the nearest CCFA chapter. You can write the Crohn's & Colitis Foundation of America, 386 Park Ave. South, 17th floor, New York, N.Y. 10016-8804, or call 1-800-932-2423. Even if the closest chapter isn't nearby, you can get on the mailing list and plan to attend some special events. A coping conference or a support group could be helpful in reducing your feelings of loneliness.

You might even want to start a chapter or a support group in your area. Ask your doctor if he can put you in touch with others who would be interested. Contact either your closest chapter or the New York office for guidelines. Whatever you do, you will want to join some chapter of CCFA to be more involved.

Read everything you can. In another column I will list some books that give a greater understanding of IBD. Meanwhile, check with the most convenient CCFA office and see what is available in books and pamphlets.

You might want to correspond with someone who shares your circumstances. The national CCFA publishes a mutual help network. If you wish to place an ad, write to: The Mutual Help Network, C/O CCFA, 386 Park Avenue South, 17th floor, New York, NY 100016-8804. Limit your ad to five or six lines.

Sometimes just having someone listen to you can be beneficial. Find a friend that wants to listen, or consult with a member of the clergy. If they are not knowledgeable about IBD, you can educate them with the available literature.

ASK AUDREY

If you are still having difficulty, talk to a therapist that is familiar with IBD. Even if there is no one available in your town, there are some therapists that now do phone consultations regardless of how far away you live. Again your CCFA or the national CCFA should have this information.

Whichever way you choose to proceed, it is important to make some connections with others who understand the effects of IBD. (See following article on Independent Thinking.)

<u>Notes</u>

Dear Audrey,

Would you please expand on the phrase "Independent Thinking" referred to in your column and include the various outlets our own inner resources can furnish us to connect with life, though we may be occasionally forced into a sedentary position. —D.T.

Dear D.T.,

It is frustrating enough to have an illness like IBD, but it adds insult to injury when others feel that, because your body is weak, your mind is also weak. Often when we are hospitalized, the nurses talk to us as if we have a child's mentality and are completely dependent. "Now *we* will take *our* bath" is a classic example. Unfortunately, after awhile we buy into the idea that, because at times we are dependent physically, we are also dependent mentally. That couldn't be farther from the truth. One of the most independent men I have ever known was flat on his back and unable to move.

Let's look at some ways we can nurture this independent thinking—ways that don't require much physical energy.

- There is always the wonderful postal system. Through letters, you can get involved in politics, correspond with someone in a foreign land, reach out to others and, in many ways, connect with the outside world.

- Nowadays, the outside world is brought to you through radio, television, books, magazines and tapes. Being flat on your back is no excuse for not keeping up with what's happening in the world and not being able to find interesting topics to talk about. Read, listen, watch!

- Don't shut out your friends because you can't run with them. Invite them to visit. Refreshments can be ordered in or brought by your friends. Be inventive: serve picnic-style, using paper utensils to make things easier.

- Write about your experiences. Keep a journal. You don't have to be professional; years later, journal entries can be enlightening.

- Learn something new. For example, you can learn a language through tapes or records.

- Use the phone. Not only can you keep up your social contacts, but you can also utilize the phone to run your house or business. Even in a sedentary position, with the aid of a phone you can shop, secure services, obtain information, and accomplish many of the tasks that you previously did in person.

- Pursue your existing hobbies or find new ones.

- If you are a parent unable to participate in active sports with your children, read to them or play games as an alternative means of connecting.

- Now that we are in the computer age, a person who is confined can expand his or her horizons through the use of a personal computer.

- Remember, just because your body is weak doesn't mean that you can't take part in family decisions and offer emotional support.

- Many organizations can use volunteers at home for calling or writing. This is an ideal way to help others as you help yourself.

Remember, IBD is a chronic illness. Although you will have difficult periods, there are also periods when you can get out and enjoy life. With a good sense of humor, an inquiring mind, and a little creativity, even this period of your life can be meaningful.

Notes

Dear Audrey,

I was unable to attend the Conference on Coping with *Crohn's* and Colitis, but I sure could use some help in coping. What did they learn at the conference? – D.W.

Dear D.W.,

I'm sorry that you were unable to attend the conference. It was an excellent opportunity to deal with the many aspects of coping with Inflammatory Bowel Disease. Although it would be impossible to capture the whole day, I'll try to touch on some of the highlights.

When we talk about coping, not only do we talk about the many problems that the disease might create, but we also talk about coping with life in general. We do not know the cause of these diseases; however, we do know that stress often exacerbates them. Therefore, individuals with IBD not only have to learn to cope with the stresses of everyday life situations, but they also must handle the stresses brought on by the illness.

I divide the subject into three parts: coping with our bodies, our environment, and especially difficult problems.

The first area, coping with our bodies, concerns doing whatever is possible to create the optimum conditions for good health. It is difficult to deal with anything if you aren't feeling well. Some actions you can take are as follows:

- Find a doctor in whom you have confidence and to whom you can relate. The patient-doctor relationship is an important foundation.

- Become an expert on *your* nutrition. There is no one perfect diet for these illnesses. However, it is important that you establish a nutritional diet that agrees with you. This can take a lot of trial and error because diets vary for everyone and can even vary for the same individual at different stages of the illness.

- Understand what medicines you are taking. It's amazing how many people abuse their bodies by using their medicines incorrectly.

ASK AUDREY

- Schedule sufficient rest and proper exercise. This is good advice for everyone and is especially important for those with IBD.

- Learn some relaxation techniques. There are many books and classes on various techniques. Find one that works for you.

- Get your emotional life together. Don't forget that the mind and the body work together. If something is bothering you emotionally, it can affect your body.

The second area involves changing or re-creating your environment to make it easier to cope. Some steps you can take are as follows:

- Make life as convenient as possible. Plan ahead.

- Carry emergency supplies with you in your purse, briefcase or car. Whether it's medication or a change of clothes, it's comforting to know that you are well-prepared.

- Know where rest rooms are. In questionable situations, call ahead.

- Check in advance if you think that you may run into trouble with your diet.

- Travel can be made easier with preparation. You can obtain a letter from your doctor, in which he or she describes your illness and its treatment and medications. You can also get the names of doctors all over the world. A folding camp stool might be just the answer for tours, etc., where a lot of standing is involved.

Maintaining good interpersonal relationships is a very important aspect of coping. Good relationships with friends and family can be a great comfort. Coping requires both being able to give and to ask for support when necessary.

I've called the third area "ways of coping with especially difficult problems." Sometimes we do everything we can to strengthen our bodies and make changes in our environment, and still there are stresses we don't seem to be able to do much about. Some of these following methods may be helpful:

- Make sure that you really understand the difficult situations in which you find yourself. Sometimes what we believe to be problems are not problems in reality. A child telling you of a bad day in school doesn't necessarily want solutions. He or she may just want to be heard.

- Use effective listening to determine what the concerns actually are. See if the difficulty actually belongs to you or to someone else.

- Find ways of problem solving that are effective for you. For example, break a problem into small parts and deal with one part at a time, or get another opinion, or seek additional resources.

- Prioritize, and put things in perspective. Sometimes we lose perspective, blow things out of proportion, and cause a lot of unnecessary grief.

- Talk to others about your feelings. Sometimes just getting them out in the open helps you to feel better. In this circumstance, the person that you talk to is important. It must be someone who *wants* to listen.

- Find other outlets for your emotions. If you can't hit the boss, take it out on the punching bag or engage in the sport of your choice.

- Re-evaluate your expectations. If you believe you should always be perfect and nothing should ever go wrong, then you're setting yourself up for disappointment and the stress that follows.

- Work on easing up the guilt and the "shoulds." They are both great contributors to stress. One of my groups gave me permission to share their "Eleventh Commandment": Thou shalt not 'should' thyself to death.

Notes

Dear Audrey,

Recently I had surgery and I'm feeling well enough to get around, but I don't feel ready to get back to work. I'm bored staying home. Do you have any suggestions?   —R.G.

Dear R.G.,

Your situation is very common. Often we are at a crossroad: too well to be home and not well enough to handle the pressures of work. I have a suggestion that will not only be helpful for you, but others will benefit as well. Think about doing volunteer work. CCFA would be a perfect place to start. To find a chapter close to you, the National Office number is (800) 932-2423. Start in a capacity in which you feel comfortable. Here are some of the numerous advantages:

- You will feel useful.

- You will be performing a needed service.

- You will meet people.

- You will be in an atmosphere where people understand what you are going through.

- You'll learn more about IBD.

- You can use this experience in your resume' when you return to work.

- You can build up your strength in a non-stressful situation.

- You will learn new skills.

- You will be working toward finding a cure.

- You will have structure in your day that is not overwhelming.

Getting dressed, getting out, and accepting some responsibility may seem difficult at first. However, you will feel better when you do. Take advantage of this opportunity to start you on your way.

Notes:

Dear Audrey,

My neighbor told me that laughter can be helpful for IBD and I was furious. She should know that this disease is no laughing matter. Where did she ever get that idea? —S.S.

Dear S.S.,

I certainly agree with you that IBD is not a laughing matter; however, let's not discount the value of laughter itself. A great deal of research is being done on the effects of laughter on the immune system. Norman Cousins popularized this theory when he literally laughed his way to health. He helped cure himself of a serious illness by watching humorous TV programs and putting himself on a regular regimen of laughing. I'm not saying that laughter could cure IBD (don't we wish it could). However, laughter provides many benefits.

For instance, when you laugh, your cardiovascular system dilates so the rate of blood flow increases. According to Annette Goodheart[1], "the laughter lady," on her audiotape entitled *Laugh Your Way to Health*, "it's like internal jogging. Your muscles go slack, you lose control." She goes on to say that many of us are afraid of losing control. That's unfortunate because, after a good belly laugh, the brain releases a powerful pain killing substance called beta endorphins which are 100 times more powerful than any morphine-type drug you can take. Haven't you noticed that your pain is substantially reduced, if not gone entirely, for the short time just after you've had a good laugh? Once we can see the value of laughter, our next step is to determine how we can add more laughter to our lives. Here are a few suggestions. Once you get started, more will come to you.

Keep a collection of articles, stories, jokes, news items, etc. that make you laugh. Get tapes and records from the library. Don't take yourself so seriously. Look for the humor in situations. Don't be afraid to be silly. If possible, attend a conference on laughter and play.[2] Put cartoons with funny sayings up on the refrigerator door, the office bulletin board or even in the bathroom.

One of the nicest aspects of laughter is that there are no side effects. It doesn't have to cost anything. It unites people, and it's just plain fun. Diarrhea, barium enemas, prednisone swelling and stomach aches can all be more tolerable if we bring some laughter to them, no matter how hard that seems. Jules Feiffer says: "You've got to laugh at yourself sometimes. If you can't climb the mountain of yourself head-on, you've got to find a flight of stairs that no one had discovered before. Those stairs can be humor."

I know you're not happy with your illness, but remember the comment attributed to William James: "We don't laugh because we're happy, we're happy because we laugh."

[1]Dr Annette Goodheart can be reached at:
P.O. Box 40297
Santa Barbara, CA 03140-0297

[2]For more information about conferences on laughter and play, write:

The Humor Project at Saratoga Institute
480 Broadway, Suite 210
Saratoga Springs, NY 12866
(518) 587-8770

Dear Audrey,

I was looking forward to becoming an officer of our PTA, but I was not asked because one of my friends said that since I had colitis it might be too difficult for me. I was so disappointed. How would you handle this situation? —S.W.

Dear Audrey,

I recently applied for a job and asked one of my friends for a letter of reference. I accidentally found out that he had written that he didn't think that I would be able to handle the job because of my Crohn's disease. I'm really frustrated about this. Do you have any suggestions? —H.H.

Dear Audrey,

Since I was diagnosed with colitis, I notice that my family is not sharing family issues with me. My daughter was having some difficulty, and she didn't even let me know. I really feel left out. Could you address this matter? —T.L.

Dear Audrey,

My friends feel that social activities will be too draining for me. Consequently I haven't been asked to any parties, concerts, etc. I know that sometimes I can't go, but it feels so lonely not even to be asked. Please put this letter in your column to let the public know that we don't want to be excluded because we have IBD.   —C.D.

I have condensed these letters and grouped them together because they all deal with a difficult problem which those of us with IBD face. Often our family and friends feel that they are being helpful by protecting us. What they don't realize is that they are diminishing us as individuals by not letting us make decisions for ourselves.

Sometimes others feel that because we are having troubles with our body, we are intellectually compromised as well. It's important to explain to family and friends what it is we feel. We have to tell them that it's important for us to retain our autonomy. Regardless of whether we can or cannot do something, we should be consulted on matters affecting our lives.

However, if we expect others to consult with us, we, too, have to take some responsibility. We have to let others know what we can do and how we plan on doing it. We have to learn to say no to things that we feel we cannot handle, and find creative ways to deal with the obligations that we do take on. Talk with the significant people in your life and let them know that you want the option of making your own decisions. Let them know that this is very important to you.

Notes:

Dear Readers,

I recently found this information and thought I would share it with you. Finding happiness despite IBD requires a whole repertoire of ideas on which to draw.

Several years ago the sociology department at Duke University did a study called "Peace of Mind." Several factors were found to contribute greatly to emotional and mental stability.

They are:

- The absence of suspicion and resentment. Nursing a grudge was a major factor in unhappiness.

- Not living in the past. An unwholesome preoccupation with old mistakes and failures leads to depression.

- Not wasting time and energy fighting conditions you cannot change.

- Cooperate with life, instead of trying to run away from it.

- Force yourself to stay involved with the living world. Resist the temptation to withdraw and become reclusive during periods of emotional stress.

- Refuse to indulge in self-pity when life hands you a raw deal. Accept the fact that nobody gets through life without some sorrow and misfortune.

- Cultivate the old-fashioned virtues: love, honor, compassion and loyalty.

- Don't expect too much of yourself. When there is *too* wide a gap between self-expectation and your ability to meet the goals you have set, feelings of inadequacy are inevitable.

- Find something bigger than yourself to believe in. Self-centered, egotistical people score lowest in any test for measuring happiness.

ASK AUDREY

As you look over these factors, I hope they will give you some ideas on how you can improve the quality of your life.

Notes

Dear Audrey,

I have always found that reading was very helpful for me. Do you have anything that you would recommend to make dealing with my Crohn's disease any easier? —P.I.

Dear P.I.,

First let me applaud your search for reading material. Those that read certainly have a head start in the coping arena. I am going to suggest books in several areas. Not only is it important to learn more about IBD, but it is also helpful to read about other aspects of life as well. I have divided some of my favorites into the following categories:

BOOKS FOR INFORMATION ON IBD

Banks, Peter A., M.D., Daniel H. Present, M.D., and Penny Steiner, M.P.H. "The Crohn's Disease and Ulcerative Colitis Fact Book." Charles Scribner's Sons, New York, 1983.

Janowitz, Henry, M.D. "Your Gut Feelings." Oxford University Press, N.Y., 1987.

Steiner, Penny, M.P.H., Peter A. Banks, M.D., and Daniel H. Present, M.D. "People not Patients." National Foundation for Ileitis and Colitis, Inc., New York, New York, 1985.

Steiner, Penny, M.P.H., Peter A. Banks, M.D., and Daniel H. Present, M.D. "The New People Not Patients." Kendall/Hunt Publishing Co., Dubuque, Iowa, 1992.

Remember that the Crohn's & Colitis Foundation of America also has many free pamphlets that are yours for the asking.

BOOKS ON DEALING WITH CHRONIC ILLNESS

Cousins, Norman. "Anatomy of an Illness." Norton Publishing, New York, 1979.

Phillips, Robert H., Ph.D. "Coping with an Ostomy." Avery Publishing Group Inc., Wayne, N.J., 1986.

Kobrin Pitzele, Sefra. "We are Not Alone — Learning to Live with Chronic Illness." Workman Publishing, N.Y., 1985.

Register, Cheri. "Living with Chronic Illness — Days of Patience and Passion." The Free Press, A Division of Macmillan, Inc., N.Y., 1987.

Wheeler, Eugenie G. and Joyce Dace-Lombard. "Living Creatively with Chronic Illness." Pathfinder Publishing, Ventura, CA, 1989.

BOOKS ADDRESSING THE MIND-BODY CONNECTION

Charlesworth, Edward A., Ph.D and Ronald G. Nathan, Ph.D. "Stress Management." Ballantine Books, N.Y., 1982.

Cousins, Norman. "Head First, the Biology of Hope." E.P. Dutton, N.Y., 1989.

Pearsall, Paul. "Super Immunity." McGraw-Hill, New York, 1987.

Siegel, Bernie. "Love, Medicine & Miracles." Harper & Row, N.Y., 1986.

PARENTING

Gordon, Dr. Thomas. "P.E.T. Parent Effectiveness Training." Peter H. Wyden, Inc, N.Y., 1988.

RELATIONSHIPS

Hendrix, Harville, Ph.D. "Getting the Love You Want." Henry Holt & Company, N.Y., 1988.

Klever, Phil. "Are We Having Fun Yet?" International Marriage Encounter, St Paul, MN, 1988.

Pearsall, Paul. "Super Marital Sex." Doubleday, N.Y., 1987.

Price, Dr. Stephen & Susan Price, MSW. "No More Lonely Nights." G.P.Putnam's Sons, New York, N.Y., 1988.

Scarf, Maggie. "Intimate Partners." Random House, N.Y., 1987.

Tannen, Deborah, Ph.D. "You Just Don't Understand." William Morrow and Company, Inc., N.Y., 1990.

GENERAL INSPIRATIONAL

Buscaglia, Leo, Ph.D. "Living, Loving & Learning." Fawcett Columbine, N.Y., 1982.

Cheng, Nien. "Life and Death in Shanghai." Penguin Books, N.Y., 1986.

Cramer, Kathryn D. "Staying on Top When Your World is Upside Down." Viking Penguin, N.Y., 1990.

Frankl, Viktor E. "Man's Search for Meaning." Washington Square Press, N.Y., 1959.

Pearsall, Paul, Ph.D. "Making Miracles." Prentice Hall Press, N.Y., 1991.

Segal, Dr. Julius. "Winning Life's Toughest Battles." McGraw-Hill, N.Y., 1986.

HUMOR

I like anything by Erma Bombeck. She has a way of making you laugh at everyday occurrences. Look in the humor section in your bookstore or library. There are many humorous books available. Everyone's taste is slightly different, but you'll have no trouble finding a vast array of books that will help you laugh.

This is just a beginning list. The books on IBD furnish much information. Norman Cousins, in *Anatomy of an Illness*, tells how he used laughter as a healing agent. Sefra Kobrin and Cheri Register share not only their experience of living with chronic illness, but also many of the practical ways of handling it. Paul Pearsall and Norman Cousins shed more light on the mind-body connection. Bernie Siegal's book is a real comfort and helps us to aspire to be "exceptional patients." We have to remember that stress does not cause IBD, but dealing with stress effectively can make matters much better. I have included *Stress Management* because it gives a comprehensive guide to various ways of handling stress, including exercise. However, there are numerous books on stress available.

P.E.T. can be helpful for any relationship. I especially like the information on the 12 roadblocks to communication. I've already talked about *You Just Don't Understand* in an earlier column. It helps us understand the important differences between men and women's conversation. *Super Marital Sex* is almost a textbook on marriage and sex. *Getting the Love You Want* helps you understand your choice of a spouse and then guides you through some helpful exercises. I've included all the books on relationships because I find that if you have good relationships, coping with the trials of the illness is much easier.

In his latest book, *Making Miracles*, Paul Pearsall comes to new conclusions after dealing with his life-threatening illness. With scientific evidence he shows the existence of miracles. Leo Buscaglia has a way of looking at life that makes you feel good. I included Nien Cheng's book on how she dealt with her imprisonment in China during the cultural revolution because I greatly admired her coping skills. Viktor Frankl shows that finding meaning can get you through experiences even as horrendous as being in the concentration camps of Germany. *Winning Life's Toughest Battles* and *Staying on Top when the World Turns Upside Down* both give excellent tips on dealing with adversity.

I'm not endorsing everything in these books, but they will give you some fresh ideas to help you form your own coping strategies. As I started to compile this list, many more books came to mind. However this should be a good beginning.

The books about IBD are sold at the offices of your local CCFA chapter and at the national organization. The other books are usually available at the library or the bookstore of your choice. Don't forget that used bookstores may also have some of the selections at a reduced price.

I also want to remind you that the libraries do have books on tape, for times when you're not feeling well enough to read. Some libraries will send you books or books on tape if you are unable to get out.

Keep reading. Remember, good reading can be a gateway to good health.

ASK AUDREY

ADDITIONAL READING

It's impossible for me to list all the wonderful books I've encountered. However, for this third printing, I thought I would add a few select titles to my list of recommendations:

BOOKS FOR INFORMATION ON IBD

Sherkin-Langer, Ferne, R.N., BScN. "If This is a Test Have I Passed Yet?" Ferne Publications, P.O. Box 16893, St. Louis, MO, 1992.

DIET, NUTRITION AND EXERCISE

Greenwood, Jan K., RDN, CNSD. "The IBD Nutrition Book." John Wiley & Sons, Inc. N.Y., N.Y., 1993.

Price, Anita L., CETN, and Allen, Linda, BSN, RNET. "Ostomy Dietary Guidelines." United Ostomy Association Publications Department, Irvine, CA, 1993.

Neilsen, Peter N. "Will of Iron." Momentum Books, Ltd., Ann Arbor, 1993.

DEALING WITH CHRONIC ILLNESS

Donoghue, Paul J., Ph.D., and Siegel, Mary E., Ph.D. "Sick and Tired of Feeling Sick and Tired." W.W. Norton & Co., 1993.

THE MIND-BODY CONNECTION

Ornstein, Robert, Ph.D and Sobel, David, M.D. "Healthy Pleasures." Addison-Wesley Publishing Co., Inc. Reading, Mass., 1989.

PARENTING

Finston, Peggy, M.D. "Parenting Plus—Raising Children With Special Health Needs." Dutton, N.Y., 1990.

RELATIONSHIPS

Gray, John, Ph.D. "Men are from Mars, Women are from Venus." Harper-Collins Publishers, Inc., N.Y., 1992.

Strong, Maggie. "Main Stay." Little Brown & Co., Boston, 1988.

GENERAL INSPIRATIONAL

Brown, H. Johnson, Jr. "Life's Little Instruction Book—511 Reminders for a Happy and Rewarding Life." Rutledge Hill Press, Nashville, TN, 1991.

Kushner, Harold S. "When Bad Things Happen to Good People." Avon Books, N.Y., 1983.

SELF-IMPROVEMENT

Jakubowski, Patricia, and Lange, Arthur J. "The Assertive Option." Research Press Co., Champaign, IL, 1978.

Simon, Dr. Sidney B., and Suzanne. "Forgiveness." Warner Books, N.Y., 1990.

Fensterhein, Herbert, Ph.D and Baer, Jean. "Don't Say Yes When You Want to Say NO." Dell Publishing Co., N.Y., 1975.

HUMOR

Don't forget the humor books. I haven't included any more because humor is very personal. However, please let me know if you've really enjoyed a particular book and would like to share it with my readers.

Keep reading. It's better than pain pills and very rewarding.

Notes

AFTERWORD

Dear Readers,

As we finish our journey together, I want to share a few reflections with you. In the beginning of the book I told you my story. During my many hospitalizations, I often wished that I would be in the position to share with others what I had learned. While this book was in progress, I became the Director of Psychological Services for the Inflammatory Bowel Disease Institute affiliated with Sinai Hospital in Detroit. My dream of being able to take an active part in the psychological needs of IBD patients has come true. Never, as I recovered from early surgeries, tubes coming out of every opening, did I think that this would be possible.

The message that I want to convey is that your dreams can also come true. I'm not saying that it will be easy, but with planning, patience and perserverence, you too can accomplish what might now seem impossible. I've provided you with lots of tools and resources. Study, search and learn to adapt. Start now to make IBD just a passenger—not the driver in your life.

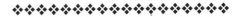

<u>August 9, 1994</u>

This is the third printing of *Ask Audrey*. A significant change is the addition of more reading material. I have found these books helpful, and I want to share them with you as soon as possible. There is even more that I want to add, but that will have to wait until the next book.

The third printing of *Ask Audrey* also adds new reviews, which I am pleased to report, are very favorable. As gratifying to me as the reviews have been, I've been equally touched by the many comments from my readers who find ideas in the book which increase the quality of their lives.

Working with clients with chronic illness and writing this book have helped me cope with my own illness. After you have read Ask Audrey, I hope that you too will find ways to increase your coping skills. Good luck. You can do it!

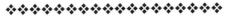

....(continued)

<u>April 21, 1998</u>

It's hard to believe six years have passed since *Ask Audrey* was written. Much has happened during that time. My newest book, *Meeting the Challenge: Living with Chronic Illness* written in late 1966 tells more of my story. *Meeting the Challenge* deals with all chronic illnesses since there are many things that all illnesses have in common. It contains more of my story, more columns and also includes a list of over 50 chronic illness organizations, phone, toll free and fax numbers, e-mail, web and postal addresses.

I have been thrilled at the response to both books. This is the 6th printing of *Ask Audrey.* It has reaffirmed that there are so many people who benefit from the information these books offer. Most of the book orders have resulted from people telling other people about it. I have heard from individuals all over the world. I am so happy that you read *Ask Audrey*, and are taking steps to improve your life despite the inconvenience of a chronic illness.

If I have helped you in any way it has been worthwhile. Write, call or e-mail your response to the book. I love hearing from you.

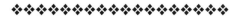

To obtain additional copies, to arrange for speaking engagements, or to communicate with the author, contact:

Audrey Kron, M.A., CGP
Center for Coping with Chronic Illness
7466 Pebble Lane
West Bloomfield, MI 48322-3521

Phone: 248-626-6960   Fax: 248-626-1379
Web: **http://www.chronicillness.com**
E-mail: **shrinka@aol.com**

*The price of *Ask Audrey* is $12. (Canadian funds: $17.)
*When ordering, add $3 for shipping and handling.
*Discounts on orders of 10 or more copies are available.

Contact the author if your organization is interested in sponsoring the sale of the book in exchange for a share of the proceeds.

To order copies of | **_Ask Audrey_** | send the completed form to:
Audrey Kron, M.A.,
Center for Coping with Chronic Illness,
7466 Pebble Lane,
West Bloomfield, MI 48322-3521

Name:_____

Address::_____

_____Zip_____

Phone:_____Fax:_____

Send **_Ask Audrey_** as a gift to:

Name:_____

Address::_____

_____Zip_____

Phone:_____Fax:_____

Please send _____ books @ $12.00 each $_____
       (Canadian funds: $17.00)
Add: Shipping and handling @ $3.00 each   _____

Total: *(check is enclosed)* $_____

How did you learn about this book? _____
_____
_____

For quantity orders please call for special prices:
Audrey Kron: 248-626-6960

To order copies of **Meeting the Challenge,** send completed form to:
Audrey Kron, M.A.,
Center for Coping with Chronic Illness,
7466 Pebble Lane,
West Bloomfield, MI 48322-3521

Name:_____

Address::_____

_____Zip_____

Phone:_____Fax:_____

Send *Meeting the Challenge* as a gift to:

Name:_____

Address::_____

_____Zip_____

Phone:_____Fax:_____

Please send _____ books @ $16.00 each $_____
          (Canadian funds: $21.00)
Add: Shipping and handling @ $3.00 each   _____

Total: *(check is enclosed)* $_____

How did you learn about this book? _____

_____

_____

For quantity orders please call for special prices:
Audrey Kron: 248-626-6960